HOLISTIC WELLNESS

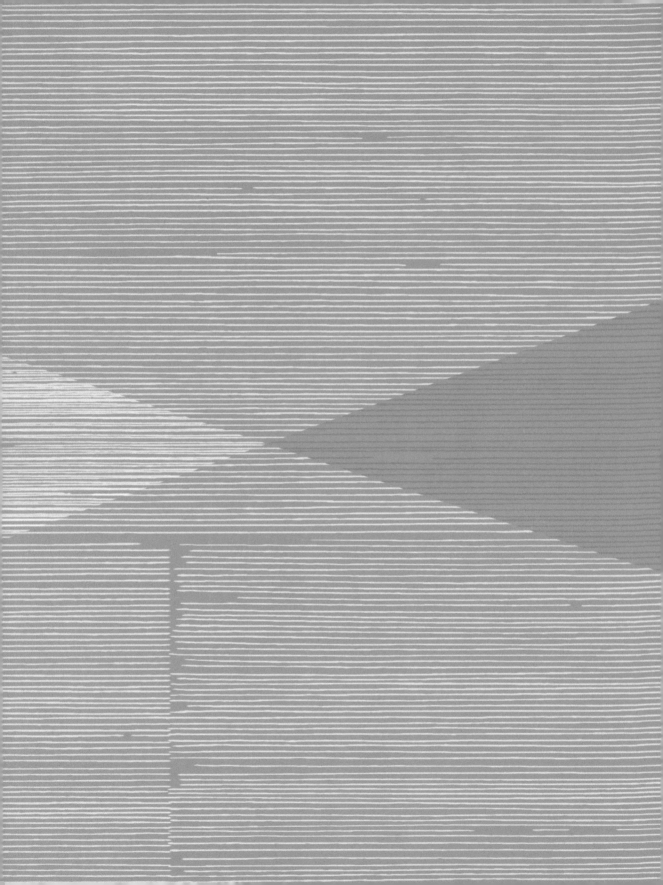

HOLISTIC
WELLNESS

Ancient and Modern Health Practices
to Revitalize Your Mind, Body, and Spirit

SARAH BAKER

ROCKRIDGE
PRESS

For general information on our other products and services or to obtain technical support, please contact our Customer Care Department within the United States at (866) 744-2665, or outside the United States at (510) 253-0500.

Rockridge Press publishes its books in a variety of electronic and print formats. Some content that appears in print may not be available in electronic books, and vice versa.

TRADEMARKS: Rockridge Press and the Rockridge Press logo are trademarks or registered trademarks of Callisto Media Inc. and/or its affiliates, in the United States and other countries, and may not be used without written permission. All other trademarks are the property of their respective owners. Rockridge Press is not associated with any product or vendor mentioned in this book.

Interior and Cover Designer: Gabe Nansen
Art Producer: Samantha Ulban
Production Editor: Jenna Dutton

Author photo courtesy of Ivan Momchilov

ISBN: Print   978-1-64739-956-6
        eBook 978-1-64739-566-7

R0

*To my mama, who loves living a holistic life herself
and introduced me to some of these concepts
throughout my childhood.*

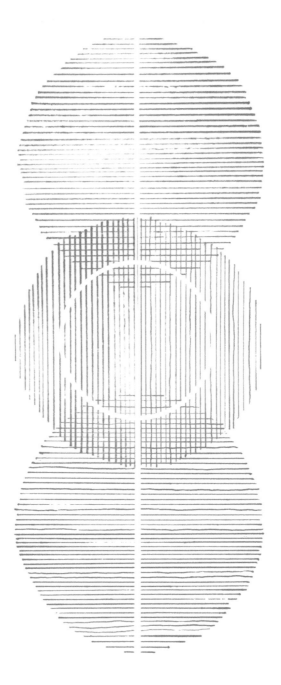

CONTENTS

////////////////////////////

INTRODUCTION

Welcome

Welcome and congratulations on starting your holistic wellness journey! I am honored to embark on this beautiful adventure with you as you learn everything you need to know about how to build a comprehensive self-care routine and health practice to rejuvenate your mind, body, and spirit. If you are looking to cultivate practices that will help you bring more mindfulness and natural ways of living into your life, let this book be your guide. Here you will find support for deep self-inquiry and renewal on many levels. I'll help you explore insights and cultivate personalized self-care routines that you can start implementing right away to nurture your emotional, physical, mental, and spiritual self.

I have been living and breathing holistic health for almost a decade and am delighted to share with you all that I've learned on my voyage. I have worked with clients from all over the world as a health expert certified in plant-based nutrition and holistic health coaching, an internationally accredited meditation teacher and mindset coach, a postpartum doula, a Reiki master, and a wellness educator. I love being an entrepreneur in the wellness space and am passionate about sharing my knowledge so that more people can experience the amazing benefits of this way of life.

Through my personal experiences, work with clients, retreats, and conferences I've led throughout the years, I have accumulated a vast wealth of knowledge of various holistic health lineages, modalities, and practices that have not only been used by civilizations for centuries, but are also becoming more and more mainstream as the years go by.

I hope you will find this book a valuable resource as you build your own holistic health practice. Treat this book as a tool in your wellness toolbox, to assist you with creating an approachable and sustainable wellness practice, even as life throws you curveballs and you evolve over the years. This book is your essential guide to keeping you connected to rituals, remedies, and sacred practices that will help you come home to your most authentic self.

I wish you the greatest success as you embark on this journey toward living a rewarding and healthy lifestyle. No matter where you are in your wellness practice, this book will support you with fresh ideas and insights from various traditions and practices. The various small steps in this book will transform your daily life, and you'll eventually be able to turn these new habits into a seamless part of your lifestyle.

What Does Holistic Wellness Mean to You?

When you think of wellness, what comes to mind? For many, the ideal "balanced" life plays on repeat in a dreamy haze of having more free time, feeling connected and energized, or perhaps feeling the healthiest you have in years. The personal definition of wellness is deeply unique for each of us.

As you contemplate your ideal balanced life, think about how you truly want to feel. What emotions do you want more of in your life? What physical sensations are you craving more of or wanting to have consistently?

When embarking on your own personal wellness journey, it's okay—and actually essential—to embrace the fact that your goals, your desires, and how you want to feel will change over time. As you uncover what makes you feel good, what your values and purpose are, and how to structure your time, routines, and habits, you will undergo transformations both large and small. I believe a wellness practice is most powerful when it's viewed as a path to personal growth.

The key is learning to adapt your wellness routines and rituals as life carries you along and you evolve. If you view your practice as a beautiful accompaniment and ally on the way, it will support and sustain you. I encourage you to think of well-being and self-care in this way. Embrace and love yourself as you are *now*, and look forward to who you will be in the future.

How to Use This Book

This book is divided into three parts to help you focus one at a time on three key aspects of holistic wellness: mind, body, and spirit. We will do a deep dive into each area, exploring how you can practice self-inquiry and self-care to nurture each one.

At the end of each section, you will read about various exercises and practices you can start implementing right away. These tools will give you the power to take charge of your wellness journey. As I like to say, a guide or healer doesn't heal you; instead, they empower you with insights and tools that help you become *your own* healer. Only you have the power to truly create magnificent change in your life through consistency, practice, self-compassion, and determination.

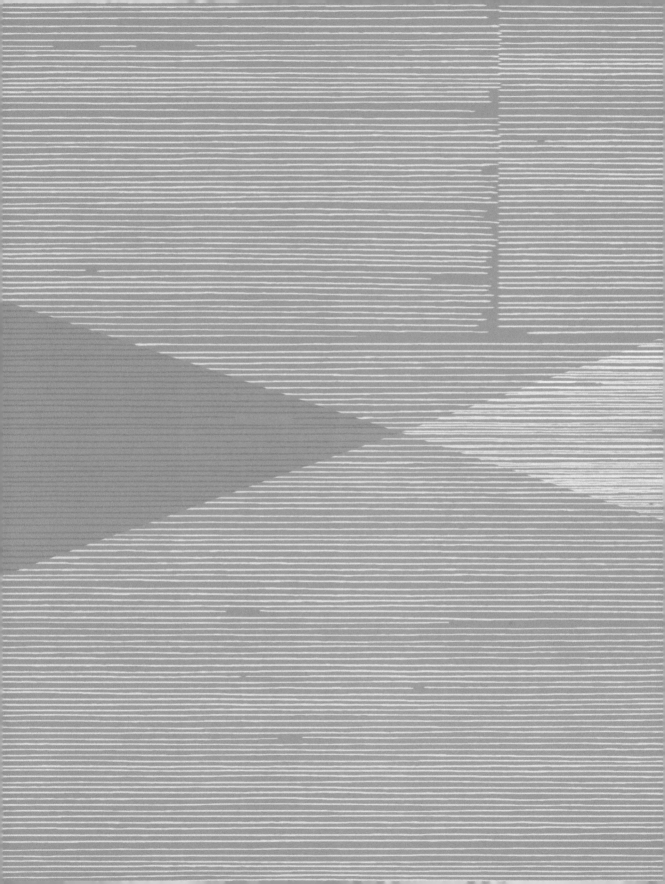

PART 1
MIND

Mental well-being is the bedrock of a beautiful, thriving life. If our emotional and mental health are not nurtured, we will not have the energy, drive, and enthusiasm to create other positive changes in life.

In this first section, we will explore various perspectives on mental well-being as well as different approaches you can use to care for your mind and emotions. By looking at a variety of cultures, religions, and philosophies, as well as modern psychology and research-based cognitive techniques, you will gain a deep understanding of the many ways you can holistically approach your mental health.

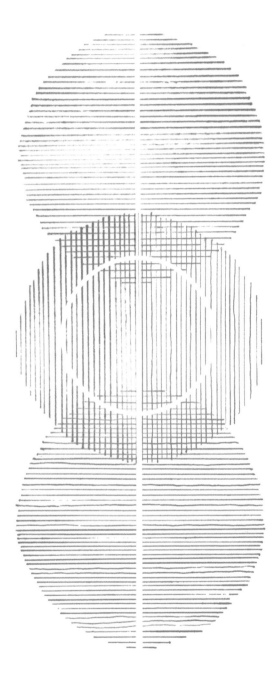

Chapter 1

NURTURING MENTAL WELLNESS

////////////////////////////////////

This chapter will explore four pillars of mental wellness, which can be used to create a healthy mindset. We will kick things off by exploring mindfulness and learning how to incorporate it throughout the day. In the second pillar, we'll explore stress in various forms and how we might address it directly. In the third pillar, we'll cover ideas from modern psychology and how to reach out for help when you need it. Last but not least, you will learn how to stimulate and challenge your mind to improve cognitive health.

Pillar 1: Cultivate Mindfulness

Learning how to cultivate mindfulness and be more present is one of the greatest gifts you can give yourself. In this pillar, you will learn what mindfulness truly means as well as the difference between mindfulness and meditation. We will focus on the numerous benefits you can get from practicing mindfulness and meditation, as well as different perspectives from various cultures and traditions from around the world.

Next, we will dive deeper into the world of meditation, where you will learn how it can level up your health, the various forms and styles of meditation, and guided meditations you can start practicing immediately.

WHAT IS MINDFULNESS?

So, what exactly *is* mindfulness? When you are fully and wholeheartedly giving attention to what you are doing in a given moment—what you are seeing, what you are experiencing, who you are with, and the experience as a whole—you are being mindful. Even though it may sound easy to do, for many it is quite difficult to be mindful in the present moment. More often than not, our minds start to wander to our to-do lists, our future or past worries, or our beeping smartphones.

When you are practicing mindfulness, you aren't trying to quiet or control your thoughts. Thoughts can come and go as you pull your focus back to the here and now, instead of fretting about the past or future. Mindfulness is available no matter where you are or what you are doing. It can help you snap out of racing worrisome thoughts and, with practice, can help you step out of overwhelmed feelings and external stressors. One goal of mindfulness is to become less reactive to challenging experiences and situations, and respond with patience and calm instead.

Mindfulness can also improve focus and productivity. When we are mindful of our thoughts and emotions, we are able to take a step back and intentionally choose how we will respond to a difficult situation.

Mindfulness can be achieved while practicing simple daily activities with focus, such as taking a walk, practicing moving meditations like yoga, or finding creative outlets like writing or painting. With practice over time, you may discover a whole new way of living!

WHAT TO DO WITH THE MIND?

Many world traditions, spiritual and philosophical, have proposed methods for dealing with the mind and cultivating inner well-being. Here we'll explore the roots of a few ancient traditions that each describe their own forms of mindfulness, meditation, and mindset in relation to the world around us.

The Vedas

The Vedas consist of ancient texts that originated in India between 1200 BCE and 200 BCE. The Vedas, and many teachings inspired by them, recommend meditation, breathwork, and mantras to live in proper relationship with our constant companion: the mind.

Composed of ancient rituals and poems and reflections on the human experience, these texts are considered sacred to many who practice Hinduism. The Vedas sparked the development of various meditation styles as well as hatha yoga and the healing system known as Ayurveda.

Vedic-inspired meditation emphasizes the need to turn within ourselves to find lasting peace instead of continuously striving and struggling to derive happiness from the world and events around us. The purpose of the practice is to become established in a space of independent joy, freedom, and bliss, which the Vedas view as our true nature.

At the end of this pillar, I will guide you through a Vedic meditation that you can practice in the comfort of your home.

Zen Buddhism

Zen Buddhism also emphasizes meditation and mindfulness as methods for actively cultivating inner peace. While Buddhism began in India, Zen Buddhism developed in China, with *zen* actually meaning "meditation." According to Zen Buddhism, understanding the meaning of our human existence requires drowning out logical thought, and it's done by utilizing different mindfulness practices.

One interesting concept in Zen Buddhism is the idea of *shoshin*, or "beginner's mind." It means releasing any sort of preconceived notions you have about life and cultivating an open curiosity instead. The name refers to the idea that when you are first learning something new, your mind is vacant and clear; it's not yet filled with expectations or fixed attitudes.

Zen Buddhists believe we are all on a journey toward enlightenment by means of looking inward. Enlightenment isn't achieved by acquiring knowledge and theories. Instead, Zen encourages us to release our fixation on the mind with all its analyses, opinions, and likes and dislikes—a compulsive pattern of chatter that could occupy us for a lifetime. Instead, we can quiet our minds through meditation to live with greater freedom.

Taoism

Taoism is a hybrid of a religion, philosophy, and way of living. Originating in China, it revolves around humans' individual relationships with nature and our place in the universe. *Tao* is translated to "the path" or "the way."

The Taoist approach to working with the mind is to focus on living in harmony with the natural order. In order to live the life of a Tao, Taoists first find their personal Tao, which is their purpose in life. Their lifelong goal is to live in alignment with this path.

Another Taoist endeavor is to release any personal expectations you have for your life. Rigid expectations can cause turbulence in the mind. Releasing these expectations helps you live in the present and escape perfectionism, focusing instead on meeting your needs and accepting both your winning qualities and foibles.

The principles of Taoism can help you be true to your authentic self, connect with the world and nature, and treat others respectfully. When living in harmony with the Tao, we naturally release anger, resentment, or aggression toward others. A combination of practices, especially meditation, helps Taoists live in rhythm with change and connect more deeply with their inner guide and intuition.

Stoicism

Stoicism is a philosophy of personal ethics originating in ancient Rome and Greece that focuses on using the mind to live in peace instead of fear or anxiety. Stoics find their path to happiness by observing the way they think about each event and moment. In a way, they were the inventors of the idea of reframing—adjusting how you see things instead of trying to alter everyone around you. This philosophy helps individuals break free from feeling overwhelmed by pain or pleasure.

Stoicism teaches that the only good is virtue, and that living a virtuous life means to release oneself from passions such as a desire for wealth, acclaim, or approval. One must practice self-control and avoid emotions like jealousy or anger, instead using reason—rather than desire—to make decisions. This philosophy also asserts that our actions are more important than our words, and that everything is rooted in nature, so society should live in accordance with the rules of nature.

Although its roots are ancient, there are many ways to apply Stoicism in the modern world. Stoicism teaches that we should change our expectations and attitudes in order to avoid anxiety and anger. Doing so means not being so taken aback or angry when a friend blows you off or a job offer or project doesn't come through—because you haven't conditioned your happiness on those things in the first place. Instead of trying to micromanage outer events, a Stoic focuses on tending to their own mind. Managing their mind and thought habits is the primary task, never controlling others or molding life to their desires. A Stoic reviews their thoughts at the end of the day, assuming that any negative emotions are the result of unhelpful thoughts, never the events themselves. Famous Stoics used these thought training practices to maintain peace in the face of exile, war, imprisonment, and execution.

MINDFUL MEDITATIONS

Meditation and mindfulness may seem like very similar practices, yet there are key differences that make them unique. While mindfulness is the awareness of *something* you are doing, meditation is practicing the awareness of *nothing* in the here and now. It's the intentional practice of taking time to become acquainted to the very present moment internally, without focusing on anything going on in your environment.

Meditation doesn't mean that you have to turn off your thoughts, because that can be almost impossible for the majority of us. Practicing meditation helps us learn how to observe a thought that pops into our head, separate ourselves from the thought, and release it without judgment.

The benefits of meditation have been widely researched and documented. One of the most notable benefits is that it reduces stress, inflammation, and other stress-related conditions in the body. It can help you regulate anxiety, improve your self-awareness, and increase productivity and focus, as well as improve sleep and manage pain.

There are countless ways to meditate, and your meditation practice will be unique to you. Here are eight different types of guided meditations that can help you ease into your own practice, which are categorized by sitting, mantra, and moving meditations.

Sitting Meditations

For these seated meditations, you will be giving your thoughts and emotions the space to be observed and will be training wandering thoughts to come back to a focal point. Let's begin with a beginner's guided meditation.

The most important thing to do before you start is to get physically comfortable. Find a comfortable seated position on a pillow, cushion, or chair to support your back and hips. If you will be sitting cross-legged, supporting yourself by sitting on a cushion will help prevent any strain in your hips or joints and can help you with proper posture.

Beginner's Guided Meditation

1. Begin by gently closing your eyes, or directing your gaze downward if closing your eyes feels uncomfortable.

2. Take a long, refreshing inhale. Hold it at the top for two seconds, then slowly exhale. Repeat three times.

3. Bring your attention to both sides of the breath: your inhale and your exhale.

4. Let your breath fill up your entire body. Gently relax and release any tension.

5. With every breath, soften every part of your body.

6. If your mind wanders, observe the thought, and then gently bring your attention back to your breath.

7. When you are ready, open your eyes, wiggle your toes, and bring your awareness back to the space around you.

You can practice this meditation for five minutes and increase the time as you desire. It's okay to feel uncomfortable during meditation. With time, you will be able to tap into a meditative space with more ease.

Seated Body Scan Meditation

This meditation is great for beginners, as your thoughts and attention will be focused on different parts of your body throughout your entire meditation practice, making it easier to keep the mind clear of intrusive thoughts. Let's begin:

1. Close your eyes and take a few deep inhales and slow relaxing exhales.

2. Focus on the crown of your head for a few moments. Then bring your awareness to your forehead. Are you furrowing your brow? Slowly release any tension.

3. Move down to your jaw and notice any sensations. If there is tension, release it.

4. Now, move down to your shoulders, letting them sink and release.

5. Gradually bring your awareness down your body—to your stomach, hips, thighs, and feet, releasing and relaxing all your muscles as you go.

6. As thoughts arise, acknowledge them, then let them float away as you bring your awareness back to your body.

Trataka Meditation

This is a gazing meditation in which you light a candle and gaze at and bring attention to the flame. This yogic meditation allows you to concentrate on one object (the flame of your candle) and is a nice alternative to meditating with eyes closed.

1. Find a comfortable space and light your candle.

2. Place your candle on a surface that's eye level to you and about an arm's length away.

3. Simply gaze at the candle. In traditional *trataka* meditations, an unblinking gaze is held for as long as possible, but you don't have to do this. Your eyes may start to water, and at this time you can close your eyes for a bit and see if you can view the afterimage of the flame in your mind.

4. With your attention on the flame, observe any thoughts or emotions that pop up in your mind, then gently send them off as you bring your attention back to the flame. Try not to focus on straining your eyes, and close your eyes when needed to bring your attention inward.

You can practice this gazing meditation for about 10 minutes, and if you feel inclined, you can continue a silent seated meditation with your eyes closed afterward.

Mantra and Chanting Meditations

Mantra meditations focus on using a sound or a phrase as your focal point. They are essentially Vedic meditations, which use a word or a sound repeatedly during the meditation practice. These types of meditations can be powerful because of the vibrational frequencies the sounds create (a discussion that could take up a whole different book!). No matter the mantra you choose, they all serve the purpose of bringing you into a meditative state and deepening your inner awareness.

Om Meditation

The sound "om" (pronounced AUM) is thought to be the sound of the universe. It is a very simple mantra to get started.

1. Take a comfortable seated position and close your eyes.

2. Breathe in a long, rejuvenating inhale. On the exhale, you will say out loud for as long as you can, "Ooooooommmm," until you run out of breath.

3. Take a long, clarifying inhale and repeat the chant again.

You can repeat this chant as many times as you like and then sit quietly for a few moments.

Affirmation Mantra: All Things Work Together for Good

This verse from the Christian Bible (Romans 8:28) is a very comforting and grounding affirmation to add to your practice. This verse explains that no matter what is going on in your life, in the end, good will come out of it. Everything happens for your unique path and for a purpose, and this is a great reminder when you are feeling stuck or going through challenging times.

1. Sit quietly and connect with the present moment.

2. When ready, say out loud, "All things work together for good."

3. Take a pause for a few breaths to let the words sink in. Then repeat the affirmation, continuing the cycle of affirmation and breaths.

You can repeat this affirmation as many times as you like, and if you feel more comfortable doing so, you can also say it internally to yourself.

Creating a Personal Mantra

A beautiful way to incorporate mantra meditation into your everyday meditation practice is by reflecting and intuitively selecting what mantra resonates with you on a personal level each day. You will need a pen and journal or piece of paper for this practice.

1. Find a comfortable space with a surface so you can write in your journal.

2. Take a few invigorating, deep breaths.

3. Observe how you are feeling today, acknowledging your thoughts without judgment.

4. Now, start writing any words related to how you feel. Try not to censor yourself.

5. Next, write words associated with how you would like to feel. Examples include "free," "accepting," or "peaceful."

6. Add one of these words to the phrase: "I AM ___."

7. Say your mantra out loud a few times, then sit quietly.

Moving Meditations

Moving meditations are another great way to tap into a meditative mindset, and are wonderful for those who aren't comfortable in a seated silent meditation or feel a bit too anxious or antsy.

Walking Meditation

Traditionally, moving meditations were taught by having students pace back and forth in a room, without having a destination. In this guided moving meditation, you will do the same, but you will take it outdoors so that you can be in nature (if you can!).

1. Find a place outside to walk in a loop without much thinking, such as around the block or around a familiar park.

2. Start your practice by standing firmly with your feet shoulder-width apart. Notice the ground beneath you and take a few deep breaths.

3. Scan your body for any tension and release it.

4. Start walking very slowly, with awareness of your feet and the earth.

5. Pick up your pace to a normal gait, and keep your gaze low to the ground in front of you to avoid distraction.

6. After walking your loop a few times, pause. Fully experience any sensory stimulations, like what you can see, smell, and hear.

Stretching Meditation

If you practice yoga, this is one of the best ways to incorporate moving meditations into your day, as yoga and meditation go hand in hand.

1. Begin in a comfortable seated position on a bolster or cushion.

2. Gently close your eyes and observe your breath.

3. Transfer to a seated lotus pose, or sit cross-legged, and place your left hand on the ground.

4. Extend your right arm up over your head and over the left side of your body. Breathe into this pose for three breaths.

5. Now, switch and repeat the stretch on the other side.

6. Return to a normal seated position.

7. Take a deep breath in and bow your head forward to the floor with your arms extended.

8. After three breaths, return to sitting upright.

9. Place your hands gently into your lap and slowly open your eyes.

KEY TAKEAWAYS

◆ Mindfulness is when you direct your full attention to the present moment.

◆ Meditation is directing your full attention and presence *inward*.

◆ Both mindfulness and meditation can help with stress, anxiety, pain management, and productivity/focus.

◆ Philosophies from all over the world focus on mindfulness, by different names, as a form of personal growth and development.

◆ A meditation practice can be unique to you.

PRACTICES TO TRY

◆ Infuse mindfulness into everything you do—such as making your bed, cooking, or playing with your children.

◆ Check in with yourself throughout the day. What emotions arise? Where are you putting your attention?

◆ Practice one of the guided meditations from this chapter a few times a week, and see which one you enjoy most.

◆ Focus on your breath more. When we are stressed, our breathing becomes shallow and short. Longer exhales calm the nervous system, and focused breathing can be done anytime, anywhere.

Pillar 2: Tackle Stress

As you have now seen, mindfulness and meditation can play an important role in regulating and managing stress. However, there are additional ways to manage stress, beginning with a better understanding of the origins of stress, anxiety, or worry in your life. In this pillar, you will learn how to decode your stress and find ways to mitigate it. There are many different causes of stress, from occupational and financial to environmental and relationship, and one or all these causes could be weighing on you.

At the end of this pillar, you will find additional stress-relief practices and tools for managing stress triggers.

OCCUPATIONAL STRESS

Even if you work in an attractive office with nice people and table tennis, stress can find its way in. There are a number of reasons your career or workplace can cause stress, and many of these stressors can be ongoing, creating long-term challenges if they are not addressed.

High Workload

When you are feeling overwhelmed by the sheer volume of work you have sitting in front of you, you are experiencing a high workload. Too much work can lead to stress, fatigue, and burnout. The good news is, you can resolve this type of stress.

First, accept that you can't do it all, and that's okay. Most important, don't be afraid to speak up. It's important that you can talk with a supervisor about your situation and look together for a solution. Seeing what can be outsourced or delegated can help you significantly. Research into top performers consistently finds that they avoid being spread too thin. They look for ways to focus on top priorities.

Conflict with a Supervisor

Another common workplace stressor is conflict with your manager. Often this type of stress can be mitigated by practicing good communication and trying to view the situation from your manager's perspective. Using accusatory language like "Why do *you* do this?" will put your supervisor on the defensive, so try expressing your concerns by saying things like "It's hard for *me* to . . ." This will help your manager see things from your perspective as well.

Another great way to handle this type of stress is by focusing on processes instead of personalities. Look for a solution rather than who is right or wrong. By maintaining close communication around an issue, you can also improve the relationship.

Process Confusion

Another common occupational stress can be process confusion. It's never bad to ask questions about a process, and in fact it can show your colleagues or manager that you are eager to do the job right. Make sure you are being extra clear about what part of the process you need help on, instead of being vague.

Deadline Pressures

Deadline pressures can be some of the biggest sources of stress at work. A great way to handle this type of stress is by organizing your to-do list based on priority. What is most important to get done? Usually if you start working on the most looming and difficult task first, it will be easier to get the rest done in a timely manner. And if you have been practicing your mindfulness meditations, you can increase your chances of staying calm under pressure. Also, breaking down an assignment into little tasks or milestones can make the project seem less overwhelming and help keep you on schedule.

FINANCIAL STRESS

Financial stress can come in many forms. From budgetary challenges to inconsistent salary, lost employment, and debt, financial stress can create headaches as well as friction in the household. But there are some proven strategies for keeping your finances on track.

Budgeting

If you find that you are having problems with your budget, a great way to get it organized is by categorizing your needs and basics in writing. For many, rent or mortgage, bills, and utilities are non-negotiables that will most likely remain consistent from month to month. These necessities always need to be accounted for in your monthly budget. Other expenses like food, clothing, and transportation can vary, and you can reduce your spending in these areas by doing things like cooking more at home, spending less on dining out, and shopping for sales instead of paying full price for clothing. The most important thing is to consistently plan a budget, and adjust it as needed each month.

Changes in Income

Another financial challenge might be inconsistent salary, especially for all the gig workers and freelancers in the world; some months can bring significant sources of income and other months, not much at all! One way to reduce stress if this challenge applies to you is to base your budget on your "slow months" so that you don't end up overspending. It's important to take care of the essentials first (rent or mortgage, bills, utilities, food) so that you know exactly what part of your paychecks are going toward these essentials and what can be saved or spent on other things.

Lost or Underemployment

Losing work can be a real struggle, especially if it happens out of nowhere. If you find yourself in a place of job and financial security, take the opportunity to start creating a safety net for yourself. You can plan ahead for potential unemployment by setting aside a certain amount of money from each paycheck for your cushion, should you ever need it. Having a plan for times of loss of income will help you feel more prepared if the situation arises.

Debt

Many Americans are in some sort of debt, with the most common types being mortgage debt, auto debt, student loans, and credit cards. Debt can feel overwhelming, and figuring out how to balance paying off debt while also paying your monthly bills can be a great source of stress. When tackling debt, it's important to get organized. One option is to list out on a spreadsheet each source of debt, so you can calculate how much money each month you can pay toward your debt. There are also plenty of debt-management tools online that can do some of the work for you. Typically, you will want to pay off credit card debt first—but focus on any debt that has the highest interest, as it's costing you the most!

ENVIRONMENTAL STRESS

Where we live, who we live with, and our experiences in our community can all have a negative impact on our mental health if they are unhealthy, toxic, or triggering. Let's explore feeling safe and secure in your environment.

Tension at Home

If you are living in a challenging environment, it can be very hard to find the rest and restoration you need at home. Challenging home environments can come in many forms, such as having a strained relationship with your partner, child, or roommates. One way to handle tension at home is by learning how to communicate effectively, and understanding that others may not be aware of your expectations of them. Setting boundaries and understanding that sometimes you can't change a person can also help you deal with household conflict.

Commuting

A great way to handle long commutes to and from work is by practicing mindfulness! This practice is especially effective if you take a train or a bus to work. You can pop in your headphones, turn on your favorite music, and immerse yourself, or simply focus on different sensations around you in a mindful and intentional way. If you have a long drive, listening to your favorite podcast or an audiobook discussing a new skill you want to learn can help you feel like you are doing something for yourself in these "off" hours.

Feeling Safe in Your Environment

If you worry about safety in the area where you live or during your commute, there are some commonsense practices you can use so that you feel a bit more protected. When you are outside, it's important to always be alert and not be distracted on your cell phone. You can also keep pepper spray attached to your keychain for an extra line of defense. If you want to feel more secure in your home, make sure you always leave some lights on when you are not home. Also, get to know your neighbors or people in your community so you feel more connected and can reach out to others should you need help.

RELATIONSHIP STRESS

Relationships are a basic need for all humans and an essential part of a meaningful, happy life. Relationship stress can arise from misunderstandings or conflicts with partners, friends, family, and even coworkers. Though many conflicts can be resolved through effective communication, some cannot. It's important to know when a relationship can be saved, and when you need to walk away.

Foundations of Healthy Relationships

Healthy relationships are based on mutual respect, shared values and interests, and honesty. They make you feel secure and loved. Both individuals in the relationship treat each other fairly and equally, work on practicing good communication, and are able to trust and confide in each other.

 As with anything worthwhile, a good long-term relationship requires some healthy effort. Negative aspects of the relationship should be brought out in the open, discussed, and worked on by both parties. This doesn't mean that your relationships—even your healthy ones—will be perfect. The key is that you and your partner, friend, colleague, or family member work together to create a positive connection that helps the individuals flourish. Here are some things to aim for when cultivating a healthy relationship. For simplicity, I have used the words "partner" or "friend" as examples, but these principles can apply to all types of relationships.

Trust and Honesty

When you and your partner trust each other, you build each other's confidence and feelings of security. In a healthy relationship, there shouldn't be a need for you to question your partner's every move. You and your partner should also feel that you can confide in each other and be open and honest about your feelings as well as your past and current lives.

Respect

In any relationship, it's important to appreciate each other's values and beliefs and accept each other for who you truly are. Rather than trying to change a friend's values or beliefs, listen to their views on different topics and treat their opinions with respect. When disagreements arise, address them in a nonjudgmental way, and consider your friend's perspective. Conflict is actually healthy in relationships, as it helps both parties work on effective communication skills. If you both can address disagreements with respect toward each other, it will make your relationship that much stronger.

Mutual Support

Another great characteristic of a healthy relationship is that both you and your partner support each other's interests and hobbies outside the relationship. You should feel like you have room to be independent where you want to be, whether that's allowing enough time for friends, for alone time, or for you to work on your passions or hobbies. There should be mutual support for each other's goals and dreams.

Admitting When You're Wrong

It can be tough for all of us to admit when we've done something wrong. In a healthy relationship, each party should be able to say they are sorry and own their actions when they've made a mistake. When you or a loved one make a mistake in a relationship, it's very important to apologize sincerely and take ownership of a mistake, as this will go a very long way.

Recognizing Unhealthy or Harmful Patterns

Relationships can sometimes become unhealthy. If you find yourself in a toxic or harmful relationship, you should feel empowered to ask for change, to overhaul the relationship, or to exit. Only *you* know if a relationship is worth saving.

Toxic relationships come in many forms. One important element to consider is control. If you think you may have a controlling partner, or if you think you may be controlling yourself, there are symptoms to watch for. A controlling or narcissistic partner:

◆ May try to dictate who you spend time with, where you go, and what you are doing

◆ Belittles your opinions or even your dreams

- Has a hard time empathizing with you or other people in general

- Pressures you to live a certain way

- Manipulates and gives ultimatums

- Puts you down or uses your insecurities against you

Psychological and emotional abuse can do just as much harm as physical abuse. If being with your partner has become stressful or if you have less freedom, enthusiasm, and confidence now than before you met your partner, your relationship may need some consideration.

Physical abuse, no matter how slight, is illegal and should not be taken lightly. It may start with verbal abuse or a slight shove and then escalate over time. If your partner experiences explosive angry episodes or threatens you, please ask for help. Often relationships like this cannot be healed, and it's important not to normalize this treatment or make excuses for behavior that could become truly dangerous. There are numerous organizations that can provide assistance. See the Resources section on page 128 for some organizations that can offer help.

Remember to love yourself. Empowering yourself to stand up for what is right, walking away, and getting assistance if needed are all forms of self-care. To leave a toxic relationship is to put yourself first, and to think of your future and your precious time on this planet.

Sexual Stress in Relationships

Sex can be a major source of stress in a relationship, especially when negative self-image and fraught or complicated views on sex are involved. In a world saturated with negative messages from the media and society around sexual expression and body image, it's no wonder sex can be a source of anxiety—and one that can affect anyone, no matter their gender or sexual orientation.

Many women, in particular, develop insecurities because of negative messaging in the media or from others about both female sexuality and how female bodies "should" be—including how women should age. These shaming messages can damage a person's body image and relationship with sexuality.

Social media has exacerbated this issue, as people present curated images of their "perfect" lives online. Although their intentions may be innocent, the situation invites comparison and can open the door to self-criticism.

Meanwhile, how we feel in our bodies significantly influences how we behave toward others. Not feeling secure and comfortable in your body can even add to anxiety around physical touch as well as reduced arousal. Insecurities surrounding body image can affect people of all genders and sexual orientations. This type of insecurity can start in childhood, especially if the sexuality you identify with is not validated by society or your community. Many LGBTQ+ individuals specifically struggle with not having their sexuality and/or gender expression validated as they grow up, in part because of lack of education and inclusion in sex ed courses.

Studies have shown that sexual education that excludes gender minorities can have a very negative impact on young people's mental health, leading to anxiety and even suicidal thoughts. Simply put, your sexuality and gender expression are valid, and you deserve to have a happy and fulfilling sex life free from anxiety and stress.

So, how do we go about improving our sexual wellness? To start, communication—as with everything—is key! The more open and honest you can be with your family, friends, and partner about sex and your views of yourself, the more positive your self-image will become.

KEY TAKEAWAYS

- Look for ways to address stress at its root, in addition to practicing mindfulness and meditation.

- Honing your communication skills is key to navigating conflict in all relationships.

- Mutual respect, honesty, and open dialogue are elemental to healthy relationships.

- If you feel as though you are in a toxic relationship, it's important to seek help and feel empowered to leave if necessary.

- To prevent work stress, try being more open and proactive in your communication with your colleagues and supervisors.

- Set a time each month to organize your finances and create a budget for the month ahead.

- Don't expect the people you live with to know your expectations of them unless you tell them. Set aside time with someone important to you to discuss any concerns you have about the relationship.

- Try being an active listener next time you and your partner get into a disagreement. Instead of reacting to what they are saying, try paraphrasing what they said back to them to ensure you understand it fully and that you are both on the same page.

Pillar 3: Be Your Own Best Freud

The amazing thing about mental wellness is that there are countless approaches to understanding yourself on a deeper level. Modern psychology is full of empirically backed insights and actionable ways we can improve our mental health and well-being.

This pillar will teach you how to apply positive psychology—specifically the growth mindset—to develop a healthy outlook that can help you work through challenges or obstacles you may come across in your life. You will also learn about tools for tapping into subconscious thought patterns and discuss therapeutic options for mental and emotional wellness.

POSITIVE PSYCHOLOGY AND GROWTH MINDSET

Positive psychology is a scientific field that studies our behaviors, feelings, and thoughts, offering research-based guidance on how we can focus on our strengths over our weaknesses. This field encourages us to live our lives in a way that promotes our own growth and satisfaction. Proponents of positive psychology encourage us to work on our own mindset in order to cultivate more joy, love, and optimism.

One of the most influential tenets of positive psychology is the concept of a "growth mindset." Reminiscent of the Stoic philosophy we already covered, growth mindset teaches that in any goal, journey, or life experience, it is your mindset that either makes or breaks your success. If you have beliefs about yourself that are limiting—such as believing you'll never learn a new skill, find love, or reach a career milestone—this mindset itself can be a roadblock to achieving what you want.

On the other hand, if you continuously shift your beliefs from stuck to expansive, believing you are capable of growing, changing, and achieving your goals, doing so can create abundance for you in your career and your personal life.

The term "growth mindset" (and its converse, "fixed mindset") were coined by Dr. Carol Dweck. Dweck studied students' beliefs and perspectives about their failures, and her research concluded that when people are in a fixed mindset, they make assumptions about what they are capable of, thus creating limiting beliefs about themselves and holding themselves back from success. People in this mindset may believe that their creative abilities, intellect, or personality cannot be meaningfully changed or improved.

Alternatively, a growth mindset is one that questions and overturns these limiting beliefs. People with a growth mindset see themselves as works in progress, always capable of development and change, with a focus on action and personal effort rather than innate qualities. Failures are viewed as lessons to be learned, which help us work through obstacles we come across in our personal and professional lives.

By cultivating a growth mindset, you will start to realize that your beliefs can evolve and change, and that your character can develop. With effort, new skills can be formed and wisdom can be attained. Challenges will no longer be scary things to avoid because of fear of being embarrassed or rejected by others, but rather be viewed as new experiences that can help you evolve into your better self in order to live a more fulfilling life. This mindset can also diminish your fear of failure.

So, how can you go about practicing the growth mindset? Here are some ways to get started:

Accept and own your imperfections. Everyone, and I mean *everyone*, has imperfections. It is what makes us all unique and human and is an important aspect of ourselves to study as we commit to our own growth.

View challenges as opportunities. When you face a roadblock, you are forced to strategize and create solutions. View these moments as opportunities to try new strategies or gain new insights about yourself, your character, and how you can adapt to situations.

Look at failure as a teacher. Even scarier than challenges is the potential to fail. If you are terrified to fail at something, try practicing reframing. Reframing involves pausing to look out how you're describing something to yourself. How are your own thoughts shaping your experience, and how could you look at that experience differently? Instead of viewing failure as an embarrassing and catastrophic event, try seeing it as an essential learning moment that is *needed* in order to achieve success.

Be mindful of the words you choose. We all have moments when self-talk becomes negative, and this habit can be harmful to cultivating a growth mindset. Instead, practice positive self-talk by replacing words like "failure" and "challenge" with "training." Another tactic when negative self-talk bubbles up is to ask yourself if you would talk this way to a friend. Treat yourself like you would treat a loved one: with support and compassion.

Find your purpose. Finding your purpose and having a growth mindset go hand in hand. Take a moment to meditate or contemplate on what you want for your life right now. When you uncover your purpose, it will be the catalyst that will develop your growth mindset, because now you have something you are passionate about to use as fuel for your self-improvement journey.

Fixed vs. Growth Mindset

The following table includes some common fixed beliefs that may pop up in your head, as well as suggestions on how you can transform them into growth mindset beliefs.

FIXED	GROWTH
This is so hard, I feel like quitting!	This is challenging, but I will learn what it takes to make it happen!
There's no way I can fix this situation.	What little steps can I take to slowly mend this mistake?
I will never be good at public speaking.	I haven't yet mastered the skill of public speaking.
I'll never be as successful as they are.	How can I learn from their success?
It's so hard for me to lose weight, I feel like it will never happen!	What are two small healthy eating habits I can add to my day?
I feel like I completely failed.	This didn't work, so what other strategy can I use?
I am just not good at this.	I can learn how to do anything I put my mind to.
I can't believe I received this criticism for my work.	What can I learn from this feedback?

ADDRESSING THE SUBCONSCIOUS MIND

The growth mindset and positive psychology emphasize the importance of working on our conscious habits, thoughts, and beliefs about ourselves. But what about our subconscious? Many of our behaviors and feelings stem from our subconscious beliefs. So, how do we access or understand them? One insightful concept that can help you tap into these life narratives is archetypes.

Archetypes may seem complex, but they are essentially patterns of behavioral and psychological energy that showcase our collective consciousness as humans. These energies are expressed through our actions, feelings, beliefs, and thoughts and can range from healing, uplifting forms to darker and fearful expressions. Studying these instinctual energies can help us understand certain themes and chapters of our lives as constructive paths to personal growth.

According to psychologist Carl Jung, who created the concept of archetypes, these energies influence our behaviors without us fully knowing it, because we hold them deep within our thought patterns and emotional landscapes. Jung believed that these subconscious impulses stemmed from a collective human experience, a reflection of our ancestral roots.

Archetypes are also found all over the world—in myths, fairy tales, and religious stories as well as in media, marketing, and advertising, and even in our dreams—supporting the notion that archetypes are universal to our experience as humans.

From a holistic wellness perspective, the various archetypes can help us understand the impulses that guide our life choices and decisions. Studying archetypes gives us another tool for practicing self-inquiry and reflection. They can help us understand the basis of our own motives and personalities as well as those around us. We also embody many different archetypes throughout our life journey. All your relationships have an archetypal pattern, and when you can start to observe and recognize the different archetypes you embody, you will get better acquainted with the various dimensions of your personality and learn how to work on yourself and evolve. The following five common archetypes can symbolize painful, healing, nurturing, and prosperous chapters in your life. I encourage you to do further research on these archetypes if any of these deeply resonate with you and inspire you to learn more about the various layers of your current disposition.

The Victim

The Victim is an archetype that we may all relate to or embody at some point in our lives. When we are in a state of fear or experiencing adversity that is out of our control, the Victim mentality can arise. It can be triggered by injustice, guilt, rejection, inequality, or personal violation. It also may come about when you are experiencing disease or illness, and you feel like you've lost control over your health.

If this archetype is a constant energy in your life, you may feel as though everyone is always out to get you, and circumstances are never your fault. Or you may believe that you don't deserve success or that life is simply unfair. You may also know people who are frequently embroiled by the Victim archetype, as they have many complaints, woes, wounds, grudges, or grievances that they dwell on.

However, note that we all have this archetype within us, and it's okay. Don't feel bad if you struggle with the Victim. It's simply good to be aware of times when this pattern is gaining energy within you so that you can move from an unconscious to a conscious relationship to it. By acknowledging that you are currently embodying this archetype, you can then take some time to contemplate and reflect on the root cause of this state of being. It's important to understand that when you become the Victim, you are giving away your power. In order to take back your power, it's crucial to stand up for yourself, speak up, and get into action instead of festering in your negative feelings.

The Mother

The Mother archetype nurtures and tends to others. The Mother is the protector and giver of life and expresses devotion and unconditional love. This protective and accepting energy shows strength and balance between masculine and feminine energies and is not tied to any particular gender. It is also not tied to the literal act of becoming a mother. Like the other archetypes, we all have this archetypal energy in our mental landscape.

When you embody the Mother, it is not only a role you may take on, but it also symbolizes the action you take. You can mother friends and family by showing unconditional love and helping them through tough times. You can mother all your relationships through acts of guidance, protection, care, and encouragement. You can even mother your work or your projects as you create them and introduce them to the world.

Additionally, whenever there is something we are "birthing," creating, or sharing with the world, the Mother archetype gets triggered. These things could be new businesses, new homes, or anything you are showcasing that is new to you and wasn't in existence until *you* created it.

One pitfall of the archetypal energy of the Mother is that it can trigger excessive worrying, fear of the uncertain, and a need to control. This energy emphasizes protection, and because it carries the pressure of growing and caring for something or someone, it is important to become aware of any anxiety triggers and find healthy ways to cope and manage them.

The Healer

The Healer archetype tends to others' wounds, both physical and emotional. This archetype can manifest in many different ways. If you embody the Healer archetype at any given point, you may take on a serious role that has an air of power behind it. In modern times, doctors, therapists, holistic health practitioners, and many individuals in the health and wellness space carry the Healer archetype with them.

The Healer helps others journey through painful situations and in many cases acts as the catalyst for healing, transformation, and better health. Different variations of the Healer have different approaches to working with pain, whether it's learning how to sit with and live with pain, viewing pain as a challenge for positive self-growth, or completely eliminating the pain with their talents.

Healer energy can be useful when you find yourself called to help others going through significant challenges like grief, personal upheaval, divorce, addiction, or illness. The Healer can help you support others but can also be called upon to nurture your own self-care.

The Alchemist

The Alchemist has the unique capability to transform and manifest goals into realities. This archetype is charismatic and draws others to them. The outlook of the Alchemist is very optimistic and encouraging, believing that anything is possible and with work anything can be achieved. There is always a strong desire to create and manifest, and a strong connection between following their instinct and tapping into their intuition.

Cultivate your inner Alchemist energy when you want to create powerful changes around you and inspire others to take action. When you create and attract what you want, you more easily connect with your purpose, and this energy radiates outward and influences those around you. The Alchemist does not see limits, only possibilities.

The Hermit

The Hermit archetype carries older, wise energy. This archetype usually depicts someone with vast wisdom who prefers living alone but also loves to connect with and guide others. The Hermit energy embodies guidance, knowledge, self-reflection, and a connection to the natural world.

Hermit energy has a passion for being a lifelong student and an interest in creating collective change. The Hermit can show up when we are in periods of self-discovery or continuing education and are experiencing an influx of new knowledge or wisdom. We may want this time to focus on ourselves and live in a private manner, and when we are ready we will reappear to share what we've cultivated with others. This archetype also comes to us as the seasons change and can be triggered in the wintertime when we have the natural inclination to turn inward and slow down.

ASKING FOR HELP: HEAL AND GROW WITH THERAPY

As you contemplate and reflect on how you can care for your mind through archetypes and positive mindsets, there may be times when you come across thoughts and beliefs that make you feel stuck or that you cannot work through yourself. Strong emotions like grief, as well as health conditions such as depression and anxiety, can be very difficult to grapple with alone. Working with a mental health professional not only helps you understand what you are going through, but also unburdens you from heavy emotions and protects your overall health.

There are many different reasons someone may want to explore therapy. You may be experiencing bouts of depression or anxiety. Or perhaps you are constantly feeling overwhelmed, which can lead to chronic stress and burnout. Another reason to explore therapy may be chronic fatigue, which usually stems from emotional issues and feelings like anger or resentment. These issues can manifest in losing interest in activities you once loved as well as periods when you feel like you want to retreat and withdraw from others.

When you seek therapy, you will learn actionable ways to work on your emotions and beliefs in order to reach the goals you set for yourself. You may learn things about yourself that can be uncovered only through conversations with an unbiased and professionally trained therapist. Therapy can help you uncover different perspectives on your life, thus improving your relationship with not only yourself but also everyone else in your life.

The following are a few common therapeutic styles. If any of these therapies reso- nates with you, seek out a therapist who is trained in that style.

Behavioral Therapy

Behavioral therapy is very action-oriented and focuses on ways to change reactions or patterns in behaviors. The theory behind this style is that behaviors are formed from past experiences, and when we focus on breaking behavioral patterns, we can then release old behaviors and reactions and learn new ways of thinking. The most popular form of behavioral therapy is cognitive behavioral therapy, or CBT.

CBT focuses on eliminating unhealthy thought patterns and behaviors through a series of techniques aimed at bringing awareness to these issues. These techniques include learning how to notice when our thoughts may be distorted or not rooted in facts, and learning how to pinpoint and identify what thoughts or emotions are triggering unhealthy behaviors. CBT can help you practice intentional skills toward behavioral change in small steps, and can be useful for those who are experiencing anxiety, anger, panic attacks, addiction, or phobias.

Humanistic Therapy

Humanistic therapy puts the focus on the person receiving therapy, so they can better understand and process their own beliefs and emotions, with the therapist encourag- ing them to do the majority of the talking. Therapists who use this form of therapy will support and guide their client without telling them their analysis or interpretation of their feelings.

A common approach to this type of therapy is called person-centered therapy. This therapeutic style focuses on having the client take the lead in conversations to uncover their own solutions to their problems. This type of therapy guides us to connect with what we know deep down is best for ourselves.

Existential therapy is another approach that can help us understand our own responsibility for our choices. This approach helps us challenge our own viewpoints and explore other ways of thinking.

Integrative Therapy

Integrative therapy is a progressive therapy style in which the therapist will create their own approach based on the client's spiritual beliefs, unique characteristics, and preferences. Integrative therapists understand that we are all individuals and react to various methods in different ways. This therapy style is very holistic and focuses on mind, body, and spirit. It can be used with multiple therapy techniques and methods in order to create a highly curated experience for each client.

KEY TAKEAWAYS

- Positive psychology and a growth mindset can help you navigate setbacks and challenges by shifting your mindset.

- Archetypes are a useful tool for identifying certain mental and emotional patterns.

- Working with a therapist can be a powerful and highly customizable tool for self-discovery and growth.

- Therapy styles are diverse and customizable.

PRACTICES TO TRY

- Write down any challenges or obstacles you may be facing right now. Then, next to each challenge, practice self-talk from a growth mindset and write down how you can view these challenges as steps toward action.

- Research different archetypes (there may be hundreds!) and reflect on which ones you embody frequently. Study the characteristics and obstacles that they feature. What can you do to work with and understand yourself through the archetypes you identify with?

◆ Consider therapy as an opportunity for personal growth, renewal, and healing. Take the time to find someone you can relate to and who is trained in specific techniques that speak to you.

Pillar 4: Keep Learning

Just as we go running, practice yoga, or head to the gym to maintain our physical health, our mental and emotional health also need care in the form of stimulation. Mental stimulation is a huge factor in maintaining mental wellness and preventing cognitive disease. No, this doesn't just mean doing brainteaser games; instead, find daily practices you can incorporate into your life that make you feel challenged and mentally revived. When we are constantly learning new things, continuing our education, exploring new ways of thinking, taking up interesting hobbies, and enjoying the arts, we are helping bolster the health of our brains so that we can stay sharp and retain good memory as we age.

In this pillar, I will show you the various ways you can challenge your mind to improve emotional and cognitive health, from research to actionable ways to get started. Just by reading this book and learning something new, you are helping your cognitive wellness!

CHALLENGING THE MIND FOR COGNITIVE HEALTH

When we are learning a new skill, reading an interesting book, or exploring a new hobby, it not only helps us feel satisfied and accomplished, but research shows that it also improves our cognitive health, both in the short and long term!

When you learn a new skill, neurons in your brain become stimulated and new neural pathways form, helping you process more information at a quicker rate, so the area of your brain that is associated with improved performance increases in density. When you learn, you are also stimulating the growth of new brain cells (yes, you can grow new brain cells well into adulthood!). You may also experience a surge of dopamine, which is a rewarding feel-good chemical naturally produced in the brain.

The best way to take advantage of this "exercise for the brain" is to get out of your comfort zone and learn how to do something that is completely unfamiliar to you. Researchers at the University of Texas studied a group of 200 older individuals who picked up new hobbies or skills to learn and practiced these new skills for 15 hours a week for a duration of three months. The results showed that there was a significant improvement in their memory retention, even a year after the study was conducted. The most interesting finding was that those who had the highest memory retention were individuals who took up the most challenging new hobbies, such as photography and Photoshop.

So, reading novels or doing your favorite crossword puzzle are great pastimes, but the key to really improving cognitive health is to challenge the brain by doing something new. When you learn how to play a sport or explore a new art technique, you are using different parts of your brain and more specific thought processes. Even more important is the time spent learning something unfamiliar: The more you work at a skill set, the more your brain will benefit.

Certain hobbies, such as learning to play a musical instrument, can also have a great impact on lowering the risk of dementia. This is because skills that use a vast range of different parts of the brain, such as the motor and sensory systems used while playing an instrument, contribute to the formation of new neural pathways, creating extra resilience against dementia and improving cognitive health in general.

For those who love reading or playing board games, there are still benefits to keeping up with these activities when it comes to preventing dementia, as long as you consistently do them. Anything you can do to keep mentally challenging yourself on a regular basis will help keep your memory sharp for life.

STIMULATING THE INTELLECT FOR MENTAL HEALTH

In the journey to create and maintain a robust life filled with satisfaction, emotional gratification, and mental wellness, intellectual stimulation plays a major role. When we explore new ideas, concepts, and hobbies, we are nurturing not only healthy life experiences, but also the health of our brain over the long term!

One incredibly rewarding way to stimulate your intellect is through the arts. Did you know that there is a whole therapy technique that uses art to help treat issues such as anxiety and depression? Art, when applied in a therapeutic setting, can be used to help process emotions when you can't seem to find the words. But you can also experiment with the arts in the comfort of your own home.

Journaling, scribbling, coloring, scrapbooking, or any other type of activity that helps you utilize your creative thinking can help you with self-expression, self-reflection, and communication. Studies show that making art releases the feel-good hormone dopamine. Even going to galleries or observing the artwork of others can help you feel inspired and uplifted, and of course can intellectually stimulate your brain.

In addition to exploring art in its various forms—including through music and theater as well as fine arts and crafts—you can also stimulate your intellect by meeting people outside your normal circle, having interesting conversations, and learning about things that are outside your comfort zone. If you meet new people while also exploring a new hobby or learning something new, even better!

Not only do these experiences help stimulate your brain, but they also help you feel more connected and satisfied. When immersed in cultural activities or amid new groups of people, you may feel happier and more well-rounded, and it's a great way to get your mind off technology and media and into the beauty of all there is to create and enjoy in the physical world.

BECOMING A LIFELONG STUDENT

So, how can you put these practices to work? The best part of this pillar is the realization that you never have to stop learning. You can become a lifelong student in many ways, such as learning something new at home like cooking, home improvement, or gardening. Signing up for continuing education courses online or at a local college or studying a new language can also keep your learning momentum going. Even physical pursuits like learning a new sport can help stimulate your brain as you are learning the ins and outs of how to play and move in different ways.

Not only does learning help with cognitive health, but it also gives you something to look forward to after a hard day's work. It can also be a wonderful creative outlet, and help satisfy your passions and add to your life's purpose. It's exciting when you realize there is limitless learning and growing in your future.

One of my favorite ways to learn something new is to attend a "paint and sip" class. It's a great opportunity to learn a new art medium while also spending time with friends or meeting new people. Another great option is taking a dance class. Listening to music can have a lot of great benefits for your brain. When you listen to music, especially soothing music, your autonomic nervous system (responsible for helping us feel calm) gets stimulated. So taking up a ballet class for beginners can be a great way to relieve stress, get a physical workout, *and* challenge your mind, while you learn a new way of moving your body.

If you love to socialize and are an extrovert by nature, try joining a book club, taking a class at your local community college or community center, or hosting a game night with friends. These activities can also contribute to social and mental stimulation through good conversations as well as learning. If you love your alone time or tend to be more introverted, activities like exploring your local museum, seeing a play solo, or taking online classes are great ways to connect with yourself and your passions while learning and evolving. Even gardening uses brain power, because you'll be learning about how to keep various plants and flowers alive and thriving. No matter which pursuit you choose, you'll be supporting your cognitive health for the long run, and making a great contribution to your overall wellness.

KEY TAKEAWAYS

- Learning new hobbies or skills not only helps train your brain but can also make you feel more fulfilled, happy, and connected.

- Challenging your mind helps improve memory, strengthens your ability to retain new information, and can prevent the onset of dementia.

- Getting out of your comfort zone provides the most substantial benefits for your mental and cognitive health.

- Exposure to new cultural ideas, as well as meeting people outside your usual orbit, can give your brain health a major boost.

- There are myriad hobbies or intellectual pursuits you can get involved in to stimulate your brain whether you're extroverted or introverted.

PRACTICES TO TRY

◆ Add mental challenges throughout your day, such as brushing your teeth or using your fork with your nondominant hand.

◆ Spontaneously get outside your comfort zone by taking a different route home from work.

◆ Take a weekend to discover new hobbies you may like.

◆ Look at available continuing education classes or interesting community classes at your local colleges or art centers.

◆ Peruse YouTube for different DIY tutorials. You can find literally *anything* on this platform, from beauty tutorials to cooking classes.

◆ Connect with family and friends more by hosting a game night, or having the whole family learn a new recipe together.

◆ Switch up your date night by visiting a museum, seeing a musical, or learning a new language with your partner.

◆ Volunteer! You'll meet new people (great for your brain) and give back (perfect for keeping your Victim archetype in check by focusing on all you have to give instead of what you need).

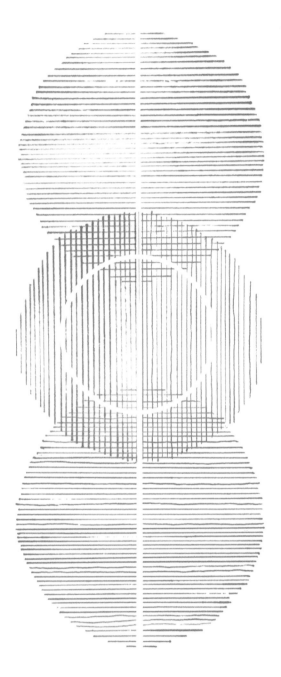

Chapter 2

DESIGN A SELF-CARE ROUTINE FOR MENTAL WELLNESS

////////////////////////////////

You have learned about the importance of mindfulness and meditation for nurturing yourself and connecting to yourself on a deeper level. You also learned about dealing with stress in different parts of your life, various psychological approaches to mental wellness, and how to study and uncover different levels of your personality. From shifting your mindset and uncovering ways to improve your self-talk to numerous approaches to stimulating your brain with intellectual challenges, you have a truly comprehensive road map for crafting your own mental wellness plan.

The following guided self-inquiry questions are designed to help you create your unique action plan for caring for your mental wellness. Take the time to reflect and provide meaningful answers that allow for deeper introspection.

GUIDED SELF-INQUIRY

» What are five characteristics I hope those around me see in me?

» What are the top five values I hold for myself and my life?

» What three things am I currently most grateful for?

» Do I belittle or show compassion toward myself when things don't go well?

» What are two habits I could change in my life right now?

» What am I doing when I feel I am in a state of flow, and how can I do more of this activity?

» What needs of mine aren't currently being met?

» Who do I surround myself with who lifts me up, motivates me, and inspires me?

» What are three beliefs I have about myself that can be reworded with phrases from the growth mindset table on page 25?

SET YOUR INTENTION

After you've written down the answers to your self-inquiry questions, take some time to reflect on what your intention might be for your current mental health. Write this intention in your journal.

CREATE YOUR ACTION PLAN

Next, I invite you to create your action plan based on this intention. It's important to remember that the wellness plan for your mind is unique to you. Use the answers to your self-inquiry questions as guidance.

A WELLNESS PLAN FOR MY MIND

Actions I will take to support my mental/emotional wellness:

Action 1:

Action 2:

Action 3:

What I no longer need:

What I need more of:

Here are my hurdles:

Here are my allies:

What I should keep in
mind about my personality
and disposition as I work
toward my goals:

How much time each day
I will dedicate to my mental
health wellness practice:

The days of the week I will
start working on this plan:

On my mind:

MY IDEAL DAILY SCHEDULE

Time	
5:00 am	
6:00 am	
7:00 am	
8:00 am	
9:00 am	
10:00 am	
11:00 am	
12:00 pm	
1:00 pm	
2:00 pm	
3:00 pm	
4:00 pm	
5:00 pm	
6:00 pm	
7:00 pm	
8:00 pm	
9:00 pm	
10:00 pm	

PART 2
BODY

Regardless of whether we are aware of it, our entire days are filled with actions that either support or undermine our physical health. Our physical well-being is foundational to living a thriving and robust life. If we aren't caring for our bodies, we aren't giving ourselves a healthy line of defense against pathogens, toxic foods, and disease. Our vitality, energy, and capability to prevent illness rely on how we care for our physical wellness just as much as our mental health.

Rather than focusing on structured routines, meal plans, or prescriptions to follow, this section should be a source of knowledge and inspiration so you can create your own plan that is unique just to you.

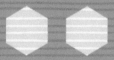

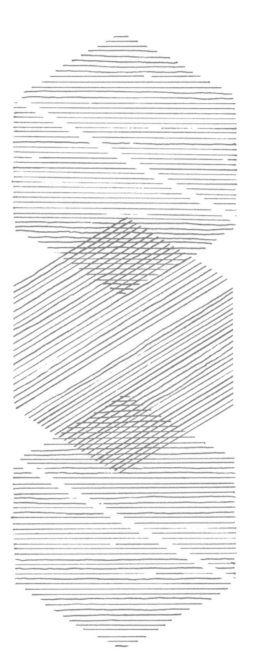

Chapter 3

CULTIVATING PHYSICAL WELLNESS

////////////////////////////////

Let's begin by honoring your unique body. Within this first pillar, we will focus on ancient medicinal practices that view our health and well-being from a deep holistic perspective. Next we will discuss the importance of eating foods that cultivate wellness, as well as how to maintain physical endurance and vibrancy from movement. Finally, you will learn about some additional supportive healing modalities that will help you feel balanced and invigorated.

Pillar 1: Honor Your Unique Body

We have all been given different bodies and have different definitions of physical health. What your friend defines as a healthy lifestyle may not align with your definition. All our physical wellness goals should be curated specifically for our unique needs and desires. This pillar will help you determine what your own wellness goals may look like.

There is no "perfect" ideal of physical health, and no finish line to cross. Your journey toward your own vitality and healthy lifestyle practices begins here.

THE ART OF INDIVIDUAL WELLNESS

Given that our health and well-being are unique, we should take a moment to reflect on the body we were born with and our life experiences up to this point. Becoming attuned to our unique needs and observing how different choices make us feel is a critical piece of the physical wellness endeavor. No matter where we are in our life path, there is room to support and evolve our wellness practice.

Ayurveda and traditional Chinese medicine are two of the oldest health- and self-care systems in the world. Both are comprehensive and holistic, focused on developing preventive practices and healing modalities based on individual wellness needs. Both require careful study of the individual and analysis of each person as a whole—taking into account our body structure, emotional disposition, energy, and many other nuances.

Thousands of years old, traditional Chinese medicine (TCM) is reflected in practices that are now familiar worldwide, such as tai chi and acupuncture. Chinese medicine focuses on how *qi*, or our vital life force (some may call this our "energy"), flows through the body. In a healthy body, the energy flows freely throughout, promoting vivacity and balance. Blockages of energy in the body can cause imbalance, illness, or disease. When working with individuals to create a wellness plan, TCM practitioners will conduct assessments to observe energy flow or any potential blockages.

TCM encourages a balance between yin and yang, two opposite energies that operate together throughout the body. Yin symbolizes the feminine, coldness, and dark, whereas yang symbolizes the masculine, warm, and light. These two opposite energies come through in the various holistic techniques that practitioners use, such as heating practices like burning herbs or using heated cups to create suction on different areas of the body, and cooling practices like breathwork and meditation.

Ayurvedic medicine, which originated in India, is another ancient health system dating back thousands of years. Just as with TCM, Ayurveda emphasizes the importance of maintaining a balance among the body, mind, and spirit, as well as the use of natural elements found in the world.

Ayurveda focuses on prevention and uncovering the root cause of physical symptoms and imbalances within the body. Instead of treating a symptom and calling it a day, Ayurvedic practitioners treat the *cause* of the symptom. Those who incorporate Ayurveda into their lives focus on lifestyle practices, including the use of herbs; specific treatments, such as massage therapies that focus on medicinal oils, herbal poultices, and body-steaming practices; and meditation or mindset practices. Ayurveda refers to our unique patterns and energy combinations as our "constitution." Imbalances in the constitution can be caused by emotional trauma or stress, physical ailments, or even the shift of the seasons. Ayurveda also emphasizes that there will always be a cycle of balance and imbalance, and the key is to understand how to work with and re-establish order when imbalances occur.

DOSHA ASSESSMENT AND RECOMMENDATIONS

So, how do we know what our constitution is in Ayurveda? What are the energies that make up a constitution, and how do they work? In Ayurvedic tradition, we are born with what is called a *prakruti*, or our baseline constitution. This consists of both our physical and mental permanent characteristics, such as the color of our hair, our subconscious personality traits, and our physical build. The three energies that work together to create our prakruti are called *doshas*, and we are all created with a combination of these doshas. As we grow up and move through different chapters of our lives, these three doshas can shift, and one can become more dominant than the others, causing an imbalance within the body. What we eat, where we live, and especially the change of the seasons can cause an imbalance of our doshas. A majority of the practices and modalities used in Ayurvedic medicine focus on either strengthening or minimizing a specific dosha to bring our body back to balance.

These three doshas are *vata*, *pitta*, and *kapha*. All are associated with our physiological and psychological selves. Vata encompasses the energy of movement, pitta encompasses the energy of metabolism, and kapha encompasses structure and lubrication. Even though we are all made up of all three of these doshas, we are usually born with a dominant dosha, and one that is the least dominant. The doshas also encompass the five elements: earth, fire, water, air, and space.

Vata

Vata is the dosha composed of air and space. It rules over our blinking, heartbeat, and breathing, and all movements within our body—even on a cellular level. Vata is the force behind the energy that makes everything from our cells to our patterns of thinking work.

Body type: A slim frame, small bones, varying digestion, and dry or brittle hair and skin.

Personality: Active, restless, and creative. Vata types are usually quick thinking, quick to learn, and sometimes impulsive.

Signs of imbalance: Anxiety or fear as well as digestive issues like bloating or constipation.

Causes of imbalance: Not having a structured routine, traveling too much by plane, too much stimulation, and too many cold foods.

Pitta

Pitta is composed of water and fire and rules over metabolism. Those who are predominantly pitta are very ambitious, competitive, organized, and intelligent.

Body type: A medium build. A tendency to run warm, sweat easily, and build muscle easily. A pitta-dominant person has a strong metabolism and digestion. Silky skin and hair.

Personality: Leaders and those with a type A personality. Can be charismatic or a bit loud and domineering.

Signs of imbalance: Skin inflammation such as acne or eczema, irritability, or jealousy.

Causes of imbalance: Too much heat, sun, or prolonged work. Too many competitive situations that promote the driven side of the personality.

Kapha

Kapha is composed of water and earth and rules over our bones and all the lubrication within our bodies.

Body type: Broad shoulders and strong, sturdy bodies, oilier or smooth skin. Slow digestion and may gain weight very easily. Their skin and hair are quite thick, and they tend to favor a lot of sleep.

Personality: Kaphas are very grounded, loving, stable, and compassionate. They may learn more slowly but have strong memories.

Signs of imbalance: Food cravings can increase and result in weight gain. Sinus and respiratory problems can arise, and feelings of possessiveness can manifest.

Causes of imbalance: Too much time in cold or damp environments, or sleeping too much during the day and not moving much during the winter season. Overeating and consuming heavy meals.

Understanding Your Dosha Balance

The following quiz will help you discover your balance of doshas in order to further understand your unique wellness blueprint. Keep in mind that many people have a combo dosha type. You may not fit perfectly into just one category.

Vata:

☐ My skeletal frame is small, narrow, and long.

☐ My skin is dry and rough.

☐ My hair is frizzy and dry.

☐ I get nervous or anxious easily.

☐ My digestion changes frequently.

☐ I am always excited to start new projects and work on them quickly.

☐ Sometimes I have difficulty concentrating.

☐ I don't like cold weather.

☐ I am very active and always on the go.

Pitta:

- ☐ My body frame is proportional and medium in build.
- ☐ I perspire easily.
- ☐ I get acne easily.
- ☐ My emotions are usually intense.
- ☐ I gain weight evenly around my body.
- ☐ My digestion is very strong and consistent.
- ☐ I like cool and dry climates the best.
- ☐ When I'm experiencing conflict, I get very agitated and irritable.
- ☐ I am a perfectionist.
- ☐ My hair is straight and fine.

Kapha:

- ☐ I have a large skeletal frame and my shoulders are quite broad.
- ☐ I am very compassionate and stable in my emotions.
- ☐ I get tired very easily.
- ☐ I tend to have excess mucus in my sinuses.
- ☐ I have slow digestion and gain weight easily.
- ☐ My skin is smooth and prone to oiliness and larger pores, and my veins are not very visible under my skin.
- ☐ I am good at keeping a consistent routine.
- ☐ I tend to sleep a lot and feel tired even after sleeping for a while.
- ☐ I don't like humid weather.

Now that you know your dosha type (or combo type), here are some tips for staying in balance based on your category.

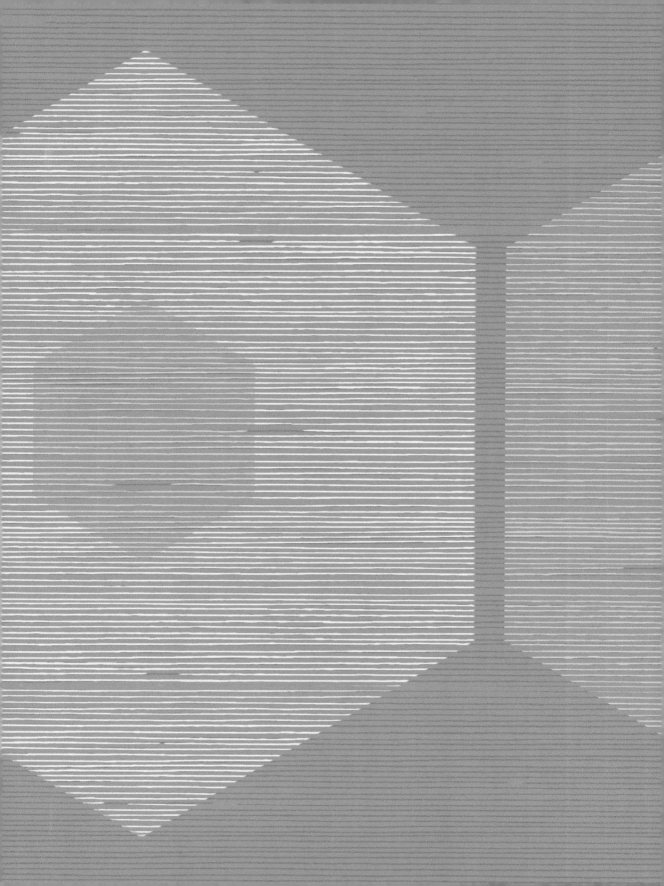

PREDOMINANT DOSHA	PHYSICAL CHARACTERISTICS	MENTAL AND EMOTIONAL DISPOSITION
Vata	· Small frame, hard to gain weight. · Appetite and metabolism are usually irregular. · Veins may be visible under the skin, and hair is dry and frizzy. · Lips are thin.	· Creative and innovative. · Mood can change rapidly without notice. · Prone to anxiety or nervousness. · Mind and thoughts can be quick and overactive.
Pitta	· Medium body build with a consistent weight. · Hunger levels and digestion are usually stable and strong. · Skin is warm and hair is fine and usually straight.	· Prone to irritability or anger. · Analytical thinker and very intelligent. · You wear your heart on your sleeve.
Kapha	· Large and stocky body build. · Gains weight easily and finds it hard to lose weight. · Appetite is steady but digestion is slow. · Skin is oily, pores are large, and hair is thick and lustrous.	· Emotions are usually stable and grounded. · Prone to depression or feeling sad during conflict. · Can get fatigued and tired easily, may experience brain fog.

LIFESTYLE RECOMMENDATIONS FOR PROTECTING BALANCE	DIETARY RECOMMENDATIONS
· Maintain a scheduled routine. · Go to bed before 10 p.m. · Avoid cold environments. · Add steam baths or saunas to your beauty routine.	· Warm, cooked foods like stews and soups. · Avoid astringent fruits like raw apples. · Include nuts and seeds in your diet in the form of nut butters. · Avoid sugar and too much caffeine.
· Avoid excessively hot climates. · Practice meditation and yoga frequently. · Wear clothes that are breathable, such as cotton. · Do not skip meals and eat at regular intervals.	· Avoid sour and salty foods. · Focus on plant-based foods and eating habits. Salads and raw vegetables are recommended. Animal products should be eaten in moderation. · Avoid hot spices like cayenne pepper.
· Eat meals in a peaceful environment. · Maintain an energetic routine involving a lot of movement. · Avoid daytime naps. · Stimulate your mind and body on a daily basis through music and scents.	· Focus on consuming bitter and astringent foods. · Avoid dairy products and greasy foods. · Avoid cooling and sweet foods. · Eat more heating spices like ginger, cinnamon, and cayenne pepper.

WORKING WITH HORMONES AND NATURAL CYCLES

When we think of hormones, flashbacks to our teen years may pop into our mind— the onset of puberty and the surge of emotions that went along with it. Our hormones play a role throughout our entire lives, affecting our bodily functions from our skin, brain, heart, muscles, and metabolism to our sleep cycles and more. Imbalances in these hormones can lead to weight issues, infertility, and physical changes like hair loss or skin problems.

Women's hormone levels fluctuate each month with the menstrual cycle and are critical during pregnancy and postpartum. Men's hormone levels can significantly impact a number of bodily functions as well. Here we'll cover just a few key hormones that influence numerous bodily functions.

Estrogen

Estrogen is involved in sex drive for both men and women. In women, estrogen is responsible for menstruation and the health of the reproductive system. This hormone is created in the ovaries and is activated during puberty to encourage the growth of breasts, broadening of hips, and growth of armpit and pubic hair.

Progesterone

Progesterone in women is responsible for maintaining a healthy pregnancy and regulating the menstrual cycle. When progesterone levels are too high, it can contribute to PMS symptoms like bloating and sore breasts, and when they are too low it can lead to missed periods. In men, progesterone assists in producing testosterone while also balancing out estrogen levels. Progesterone in men helps regulate sleep, mood, and libido. It also contributes to bone mass and many additional functions in the male body that can affect energy levels and even anxiety levels.

Testosterone

Testosterone plays a role in the sex drive of both men and women, but is primarily a male sex hormone. This hormone is responsible for helping develop various parts of the male reproductive system, maintaining sperm production, and supporting muscle mass and the creation of body hair in men. In women, testosterone is created in much smaller amounts but still contributes to muscle growth and sex drive.

The Menstrual Cycle

So, how can a woman put all this together to manage her monthly cycle? During the first part of the cycle, the follicular phase, estrogen and progesterone start to increase, triggering the reproductive system to prepare for fertilization of an egg. When women ovulate, estrogen comes to a peak and testosterone is released. During the third phase, or luteal phase, both estrogen and progesterone are high to support a possible pregnancy. If there is not a pregnancy, they both decrease rapidly to allow for the menstrual cycle to start again. The final phase is the menstrual phase, in which both progesterone and estrogen have dropped off and menstruation begins.

As these hormones fluctuate throughout each phase, they can affect your energy levels as well as your mood and productivity. When you listen to your body and your hormonal changes throughout the month, you can adapt your routine in accordance with your hormones, as opposed to fighting against them. Here are some examples:

Follicular phase

- Support your estrogen levels with probiotic foods like sauerkraut and kimchi.
- Keep movement to moderate or light cardio.
- Do more of your creative work during this phase as your brain power increases.

Ovulatory phase

- Include antioxidant-rich foods into your diet like fruits and vegetables.
- Higher-intensity workouts may feel great during this energetic phase.
- Schedule date nights and important meetings during this phase because confidence levels are increasing.

Luteal phase

- Foods that are packed with magnesium, such as spinach, pumpkin seeds, and dark chocolate, will help during this phase. Alcohol, salt, and processed foods should be limited.

- Strength-training classes can be enjoyed during this time because there is more stamina and strength within your body.

- Your energy may direct you to reflect on your goals and look inward, doing more nurturing work.

Menstrual phase

- Keep workouts and activity light during the menstrual phase when you are experiencing your period.

- Focus on soothing and warming foods like teas and stews. Limit alcohol and caffeine.

- Rest and recovery should be the theme of this week.

LOVING YOUR BODY AS YOU AGE

As we move through life, there are so many outside voices trying to tell us how to look or how to live that may not fully align with reality. Especially as we get older, cultural messages often try to make us view aging as something negative—that we need special creams or treatments for wrinkles or that aging is some sort of problem that needs a solution.

Media messaging is loud and clear: Try to stay young. These messages can play on preexisting insecurities that often manifest as we age. But what if, instead, we started to accept aging as an integral part of living a fulfilled life? That the wrinkles we get around our eyes when we smile come from meaningful, happy moments throughout our lives?

One way to reframe your thinking about aging is to focus on the function of your body, rather than how you look on a given day. Take time to intentionally appreciate what you are physically accomplishing. Focus on your strength, flexibility, or energy and celebrate all your body is doing to support you. Remember that you are wonderfully unique and that the majority of the images you see in the media are doctored to "perfection."

Aging gracefully isn't merely for the lucky few, either. Research finds that what you eat, how you move, and several other lifestyle factors shape the aging experience and actually turn gene markers on and off in the process. So remember that your DNA expression is not a foregone conclusion and family health challenges don't have to become your own. In addition, research shows that maintaining a positive outlook on life may help you live around seven years longer.

KEY TAKEAWAYS

- ◆ Each of us is mentally and physically unique, and should develop our own wellness and self-care routine.

- ◆ There is no perfect ideal of health. How you view yourself should be based on *your* own goals, not the goals of others.

- ◆ Holistic health systems like traditional Chinese medicine and Ayurveda invite us to study our unique bodies and work with our individual constitutions to promote wellness.

- ◆ Understanding the three doshas can help us tailor our health needs to our specific body and energy types.

- ◆ Our hormones are extremely important and play a role in how we regulate weight, sleep, and our reproductive health.

- ◆ Supporting our health as we age should be a part of embracing and celebrating each year that goes by, instead of trying to find the fountain of youth.

- Write down a few lifestyle practices you can add to your life from your dosha assessment.

- If you have a monthly menstrual cycle, experiment with tracking it to see if your energy correlates with the different phases of your cycle. Work with your cycle to see if your productivity and activity levels can be supported to the best of their abilities throughout the month.

- Study your digestion. If you find that you have irregular digestion like bloating or constipation, you could have a dietary intolerance.

- If you are curious, do some further readings on traditional Chinese medicine and its various holistic practices, such as Chinese herbalism, cupping, and other modalities.

- Protect your balance, flexibility, and overall health at every age by spending at least 30 minutes moving each day. Walking, housework, and gardening are simple ways to stay in motion.

Pillar 2: Eat Beautifully

Our eating habits are a huge slice of the wellness pie. What we consume can either fuel our energy and enhance our vitality or be a detriment to our health and a contributor to disease. When you focus on eating foods that are rich in vitamins and minerals, you are supporting yourself on so many levels. Eating well can help you maintain a healthy weight, increase your energy levels, and be one of the most important lines of defense against future ailments.

For simplicity, I'll focus in this section on the dietary patterns and food traditions followed by groups of people who live longer and have lower rates of disease than anywhere else in the world. Researches have dubbed these communities the "Blue Zones." I will be sharing what exactly makes the people living in these pockets of the world so healthy. We will also discuss some specific foods that can be helpful and harmful, as well as the importance of eating natural foods.

DINING LIKE A CENTENARIAN

The term "Blue Zone" was coined by journalist Dan Buettner and a team of researchers while studying longevity patterns around the world. Buettner and the research team focused on five regions in the world that have the largest populations of centenarians—people who live to be 100 and older. He has since written extensively about the many similarities among these geographically scattered groups in an effort to distill their cultural patterns into actionable advice anyone can use to live a long, robust life. Their data is quite remarkable!

Blue Zones research indicates that genetics account for only 20 to 30 percent of one's life span, and lifestyle and dietary factors play a primary role in longevity. Blue Zone residents have great social circles filled with strong human connections, are very active and walk often, are unlikely to smoke, hold their families as their highest priority, and, most important, eat a rich and diverse diet made of primarily plants.

Where People Forget to Die

So where exactly are these areas? Let's take a closer look at the specific dietary habits of these five different Blue Zones that were studied by Buettner and his group of researchers.

Okinawa, Japan

These islands in Japan have one of the highest ratios of centenarians in the world, with around 6.5 people out of 10,000 living to be 100. Their diet emphasizes eating fresh, local food, often from their own community gardens. Common foods of the Okinawan diet are seaweed, turmeric, tofu, garlic, green tea, shiitake mushrooms, bitter melons, and brown rice. Meals primarily consist of plant-based stir-fries, sweet potatoes, and tofu. As they sit for a meal, it's common for Okinawans to say over the food, "*Hara hachi bu*," which means "80 percent full." They believe it's very important not to overfill the stomach.

Sardinia, Italy

The Italian island of Sardinia is an unusual Blue Zone in that just as many men reach age 100 as women. Many residents here work as shepherds, handling livestock and roaming the hilly terrain all day. Their diets are high in goat's and sheep's milk and cheese. Sardinian diets also include fennel, beans like chickpeas and fava beans, tomatoes, sourdough bread, barley, and an antioxidant-rich local red wine. Meat in Sardinia is typically reserved for special occasions, and olive oil is incorporated into many meals to add healthy fat. Another interesting ingredient incorporated into the lives of many Sardinians is milk thistle tea, which contains anti-inflammatory properties and is believed to help cleanse the liver.

Nicoya Peninsula, Costa Rica

This beautiful area of Costa Rica is filled with sunshine and fresh air that the people of this peninsula get to enjoy daily. Not only does their daily dose of vitamin D boost their health, but their plant-based diet does, too. Nicoyans' diets are rich in corn; fruits like papayas, peaches, and bananas; rice and beans; and fresh herbs like cilantro. Homemade corn tortillas make up a large portion of meals, and black beans are enjoyed almost every single day. The legume- and grain-rich diet is minimally processed (if at all) and filled with crucial vitamins, minerals, and antioxidants.

Loma Linda, California

This community in California follows an entire lifestyle that is dedicated to health, wellness, religion, and connection. This area houses a high percentage of Seventh-Day Adventists—a Christianity-based religion—who are primarily vegetarian, abstain from drinking alcohol and smoking, and have a combination of lifestyle factors that contribute to a long and healthy life. This religion coined the term "Garden of Eden diet," which emphasizes plant-based foods consisting of vegetables, fruits, nuts, and grains, and frowns upon the killing of animals for food. This diet may sometimes include eggs and dairy, and dinner is usually eaten early in the evening. Water is the primary drink of choice, and even sugar is avoided.

Ikaria, Greece

Another island, Ikaria, focuses on specific preparations of food and emphasizes a primarily plant-based diet with moderate amounts of fish. Food staples in this part of the world include leafy greens, honey, potatoes, goat's milk, and legumes such as lentils, black-eyed peas, and chickpeas. Meat, like goat, is eaten only occasionally. Almost 30 percent of this population's daily diet consists of vegetables, followed by fruits, legumes, and potatoes. An interesting note is that their primary starch comes from potatoes instead of grains. In fact, grains make up only about 1 percent of their diet! This diet is the basis for the widely popular Mediterranean diet.

Mediterranean Diet

You may have heard of the Mediterranean diet, which has gained a lot of popularity in recent years in the mainstream nutrition and wellness worlds, as it's touted to promote various health benefits. The Mediterranean diet focuses on eating foods commonly consumed in Mediterranean nations, like Greece and Italy, with an emphasis on vegetables, legumes, nuts, seeds, fruits, seafood, olive oil, and whole grains.

Countless studies have shown the benefits of eating a Mediterranean Diet, like maintaining a healthy heart, preventing type 2 diabetes, and promoting healthy weight levels. Studies show it can also help improve blood sugar levels and fend off disease, thanks to high antioxidants and phytonutrient levels found in its foods. It's also a great, flavorful dietary lifestyle that doesn't focus on counting calories or other tedious methods to maintain a healthy eating plan.

Many of the foods found in the Mediterranean region are accessible around the world—like vegetables, fruits, legumes, potatoes, nuts, seafood, and healthy fats like organic butter and olive oil.

FOOD HEROES AND FOOD ZEROES

Wondering where to start on your healthy-eating journey? Here are 10 of my favorite nutrient-dense superfoods that you can easily start incorporating into your diet right away, as well as 4 food zeroes that you can mindfully start to minimize.

Food Heroes

Dark leafy greens. This vegetable group includes spinach, kale, collard greens, arugula, swiss chard, and dandelion greens (a popular leafy green in Greek cuisine). Dark leafy greens are a wonderful source of antioxidants, with spinach specifically being one of the highest sources of antioxidants in the veggie world. These veggies are packed with good-for-you nutrients like magnesium, iron, calcium, zinc, fiber, and vitamin C. Fiber will help you maintain healthy digestion levels; vitamin C and zinc are wonderful immune-supporting nutrients; and iron, magnesium, and calcium are essential minerals you need for strong bones, energy, and muscle recovery. You can easily add leafy greens to salads, soups, stews, and even pasta recipes.

Cruciferous vegetables. This vegetable group includes cabbage, cauliflower, kale, broccoli, and Brussels sprouts. Studies have shown that these foods have the potential to fight and prevent certain types of cancer, and they also help regulate natural estrogen levels within the body. Cruciferous vegetables are a great source of antioxidants and vitamins that will help boost your energy levels, and they also aid in digestion.

Berries. Strawberries, blueberries, raspberries, and blackberries are really great fruit choices, as they are low on the glycemic index, meaning they won't spike your blood sugar like sweeter fruits can. They are also packed with antioxidants. Blueberries specifically have some of the highest antioxidant levels of any food. When you focus on eating antioxidant-rich foods, you are helping your body reduce inflammation and fight off oxidative damage from things like sun exposure, environmental pollutants, and toxins that get accumulated from processed foods.

Beets. Beets are root veggies that pack a major nutritional punch. With high levels of magnesium, potassium, vitamin B, iron, and copper, beets support our health on a cellular level. Beets can help keep your blood pressure at a healthy level, they support brain and digestive health, and they have anti-inflammatory properties to help fend off disease. I love adding cooked beets to summer salads with feta or goat's cheese, a squeeze of lemon, and fresh basil.

Nuts and seeds. This superfood group includes almonds, walnuts, pistachios, pecans, Brazil nuts, chia seeds, flaxseed, pumpkin seeds, and hazelnuts, to name a few. Nuts are a staple in plant-based diets and are packed with digestion-boosting fiber, protein, and healthy fats. Even though nuts may be higher in calories than other foods, that isn't a bad thing! Those calories are being put to good use because your body will use them for protein, energy, and weight management. You can include more nuts and seeds in your diet by enjoying a handful as a snack, adding them to salads, or sprinkling them on top of yogurt.

Olive oil. Olive oil contains a type of fat called monounsaturated fatty acid, which helps reduce inflammation, helps support joint health, and even has beauty benefits for your hair, skin, and nails. This oil contains vitamins E and K, which help boost heart and cellular health. It's important to source cold-pressed extra-virgin olive oil, which is minimally processed and maintains the integrity of the oil and nutrients within it.

Beans and legumes. This food group includes lentils, black beans, chickpeas, navy beans, butter beans, peas, edamame, pinto beans, and more. Beans and legumes are another great source of protein, fiber, and vitamins that help support healthy weight and cholesterol levels. I like adding beans to soups, especially chili, or vegetarian taco recipes.

Fermented foods. Foods such as sauerkraut, kimchi, kombucha, miso, kefir, and yogurt have gone through a fermentation process that creates probiotics, which are healthy bacteria that reduce inflammation and feed your gut to maintain a balanced microbiome. You may be familiar with probiotics in supplement form, but these fermented foods are also really great sources that are bioavailable, meaning they get absorbed into your body very easily.

Avocado. Another wonderful healthy-fat food, avocados are loaded with magnesium, which is important in maintaining healthy energy levels, blood pressure, and sugar levels, as well as promoting good sleep. Avocados are also a great source of omega-3s (healthy fats); an assortment of B vitamins; and vitamins C, E, and K. Even though avocados may be high in calories, their rich nutrients guarantee the calories will be put to good use. The easiest ways to incorporate avocado into your day is by making guacamole or adding a dollop to your morning toast.

Ancient grains. Grains sometimes get a bad rap because many people group all grains in with processed breads and pastas. Ancient grains, on the other hand, include quinoa, farro, barley, oats, and buckwheat. Quinoa is a wonderful grain source packed with protein and vitamins. All the ancient grains mentioned here contain fiber, antioxidants, and vitamins that help with heart health and disease prevention. You can use quinoa or farro instead of pasta, and they make great side dishes when you need more sustenance in your meal.

Food Zeros

Refined sugar. It is common knowledge that refined sugar isn't good for you. Sugar can sneak up in a multitude of processed foods and condiments, and added sugars are lurking in many beverages and snack foods. When you consume too much refined sugar, it affects your insulin levels, which, when not kept in check, can contribute to type 2 diabetes and heart disease. Eating too much refined sugar may also disrupt the hunger hormone leptin, which gives you cues when you are feeling full. When you eat more sugar, it can lead to craving even more sugar, and an unhealthy cycle can form.

Processed carbohydrates. Processed carbs can be in the form of breads, pastas, cereals, and baked goods. Usually processed carbs are made from refined wheat, which does not have a lot of nutritional value and can lead to big spikes in your insulin levels. Processed or refined carbs are also digested fairly quickly, which can lead to you feeling less full and thus overeating.

Processed meat. Processed meat includes foods like sausages, salami, hot dogs, jerky, ham, bacon, cured meat, and so on. These meats typically contain dyes, sugars, preservatives, flavor enhancers, high levels of sodium, and other added ingredients that have been linked to heart disease and cancer. Eating too many processed meats can also lead to high blood pressure and digestive problems.

Fried foods. Fried foods are usually quite high in empty calories and unhealthy fats, making them a potential contributor to weight gain as well as a number of medical conditions. Eating too many fried foods can increase bad cholesterol levels and the chances of experiencing a heart attack and other heart disease. This unhealthy eating habit can also contribute toward insulin resistance, which can lead to type 2 diabetes.

LEVEL UP TO WHOLE FOODS

What do all the previously mentioned "food heroes" have in common with Mediterranean and Blue Zones eating habits? A focus on whole foods. Whole foods are foods that are eaten in their natural form and have been minimally processed or refined, if at all. Whole foods are foods from the earth that retain their natural state and do not have any added rancid oils, preservatives, food coloring, or other ingredients.

The following table lists 15 common processed foods, with respective whole foods that can act as healthier substitutions.

PROCESSED SNACKS	HEALTHY ALTERNATIVES
Potato chips or crackers	Cucumber slices
Pretzels	Homemade kale chips
Flavored yogurt	Greek yogurt with honey and fresh berries
Pastries	Whole-grain bread with nut butter
Packaged cereal	Steel-cut oatmeal with bananas
Bagel and cream cheese	Whole-grain toast with fresh avocado
Fried chicken	Rotisserie chicken
Diet and regular soda	Sparkling water with lemon
Chocolate chip cookies	Homemade coconut or oat flour cookies
Fritos	Oven-baked corn tortilla strips
Fruit roll-ups	Fresh berries, dried apricot, or pineapple
French fries	Oven-baked sweet potato fries
Chips, pretzels, or tortilla strips with store-bought dips	Raw veggies and homemade hummus
Peanut butter and jelly sandwich on white bread	Apple and peanut butter
Orange juice	Fresh orange slices

KEY TAKEAWAYS

- What we eat is one of the most important factors in our general wellness, either fueling us for optimal health or adding toxicity to our systems.

- The food we eat can affect our cognitive health and mood.

- Residents in the Blue Zones have the largest populations of people who live to be 100 years and older, and they favor natural, plant-heavy diets.

- The Mediterranean diet is a wonderful way to boost your health without following an overly structured or complicated regimen.

- Superfoods like dark leafy greens and berries provide high-quality nutrients and antioxidants that your body needs for optimal health.

- Refined sugar, processed carbs, fried foods, and processed meats should be avoided or minimized.

- Lots of common processed foods can be replaced with nutritious whole foods instead.

PRACTICES TO TRY

- Invest in a great Mediterranean or Japanese cookbook to learn recipes from these healthy parts of the world.

- Try incorporating one new superfood every few days.

- Take note of what you eat for two weeks by starting a food journal.

- Experiment with the healthy food swaps listed on page 67 the next time you're craving chips or cookies.

Pillar 3: Move Wisely

Moving our bodies is already a part of most of our daily schedules. We move during our morning routines, when we run errands, and when we do chores around the house. Some of us move our bodies daily more than others depending on the industries we work in, as well as what type of mobility limitations we may have. But no matter how physically active you are, trying to be more purposeful with your daily movements, such as adding more walking to your commute or finding time to exercise, can be yet another wonderful tool for promoting health and wellness.

When you are intentional about your movement, especially in the form of exercise, you are supporting your cardiovascular health, boosting your immune system, nurturing your emotional and mental wellness, and promoting longevity and energy. Exercise releases feel-good hormones and chemicals, supports a healthy digestive system, and is simply all-around beneficial for health. In this pillar, we will go over various forms of movement in order to empower you to create your own movement program. Remember that each body is unique. Seek out movement you enjoy and that supports the current state of your body.

CARDIO

How do you feel when you dance to your favorite music at a concert, take in fresh air on a hike, or bike along a scenic route? This type of movement encourages the release of endorphins, leaving us feeling refreshed and invigorated. Cardio is a special form of exercise that works your cardiovascular system through moderate or high-intensity activity.

Cardio comes in all shapes and sizes, from jogging or running to rowing, swimming, and kickboxing. There is a form of cardio that can work well for just about anyone at any age. No matter what form of cardio you choose, just 30 minutes of this type of movement at a time can give you health-boosting benefits.

When you are doing cardio, you are burning primarily fat as a fuel source, followed by carbohydrates and protein. One of the most popular reasons people add cardiovascular exercises to their routine is its weight-loss benefits, but the perks don't stop there. Other benefits of cardio include improved oxygen levels throughout the body, stronger lungs, a strengthened heart, better circulation, and regulation of blood sugar, as well as what many call a "runner's high," which is the result of a surge of feel-good hormones.

STRENGTH TRAINING

Some people may shy away from strength training for fear of "bulking up," but in truth, strength training can actually make you a lean, mean, strong machine. Strength training has a host of benefits that not only impact muscle mass, but also improve other areas of your physical health, like increasing bone density, burning calories, helping your joints stay flexible, and improving balance.

When you strength train, you are building and protecting your muscle mass, which naturally helps protect your joints and bones, as the supporting muscles around them are sturdy and strong. When you have strong muscles, it is that much easier to bend down to clean around the house or pick up your children or grandchildren with ease. Another benefit of strength training is that it helps boost testosterone, which women need in order to create lean muscles. And another perk of supporting testosterone levels is that it helps burn more calories, even after the strength-training session is over. Lastly, when we increase our lean muscle mass, we in turn help boost our metabolism, which dictates how many calories we burn throughout the day.

Strength training is especially important as we age in order to protect our mobility and prevent broken bones from falls or stumbles. When women age, the metabolism slows down, in large part because of loss of lean muscle mass (anywhere between 3 and 5 percent each year after age 30).

There is also evidence that increased muscle mass is associated with preventing dementia. Studies have shown that six months of strength training improved overall cognitive performance and protected the areas of the brain that are vulnerable to degenerative disease as we age.

To get started with strength training, you can find many videos on YouTube, as well as fitness studios that offer virtual classes you can take in the comfort of your own home. You could work with weights and resistance bands or, in some cases, use your own body weight. Keep it simple and remember there are many ways to build and protect your strength.

YOGA

Yoga is a wonderful form of movement that supports your mind, body, and spirit. Considered a moving meditation by some, yoga also promotes strength, balance, and flexibility.

Flexibility contributes to our mobility as well as the management of chronic pain. Yoga also helps improve balance, muscle tone, inflammation levels, athletic performance, energy, metabolism, and circulatory health.

Studies have shown that practicing yoga can lower the stress hormone cortisol, which can help fend off anxiety and depression. There are several schools of yoga. Here we will discuss three of the most widely practiced types: hatha, vinyasa, and restorative.

Hatha Yoga

This traditional yoga practice emphasizes the importance of balancing opposite forces. Hatha incorporates postures that help strengthen the different balances of the body, such as fusing together body and breath, increasing strength while also nurturing flexibility and mental calm. Hatha is great for beginners and can be considered a foundational practice for other schools of yoga, like Bikram or Ashtanga.

Vinyasa Yoga

This yoga style focuses on the body finding a flow state. Another style that welcomes beginners, vinyasa emphasizes the importance of connecting the breath with every movement. Vinyasa yoga is gentle and mindful; it incorporates various swift or slow movements while maintaining a nice rhythm, almost like a slow dance. This yoga style is great if you like continual movement rather than holding postures for longer periods.

Restorative Yoga

Restorative yoga is very gentle and nurturing for the mind. A lot of the class is designed to help trigger the parasympathetic nervous system in the body through slow movements and using comfortable props. Relaxation-oriented poses are held for long periods (sometimes up to five minutes) in order to settle the body into a state of deep calm. The focus is less on the physical exertion of movements and more on helping the body drift into "restorative" mode. This yoga style is great as a complement for those who do more intense forms of exercise and need practices that will calm the mind and soothe the body.

TAI CHI AND QIGONG

Like yoga, tai chi and qigong incorporate mindfulness into every moment of the practice. The many styles of tai chi fuse gentle movement and breath to improve the flow of energy (or qi) in the body. Sometimes referred to as an art form, tai chi features slow and steady choreographed movements designed to boost vitality throughout every organ and system of the body.

Tai chi is easy to learn and to incorporate into your everyday routine. It can be not only a physical practice but also a deeply spiritual self-care modality and moving meditation.

Qigong is another mind-body movement practice that incorporates breathwork, movement, sound, and self-massage. There are also numerous schools of qigong, and it also works to improve the flow of qi in the body. *Qigong* translates to "working with the qi," and its purpose is to encourage energy to flow freely in the body by using slow, intentional movements. Qigong employs repeated movements to help stimulate the cardiovascular system and muscles, making it a bit more rigorous than tai chi.

The benefits of both these practices are vast and supported by multiple studies. Physical benefits include improved flexibility, balance, circulation, muscle strength, and joint health. Research on tai chi has shown its benefits include helping those with cardiovascular issues. Mental benefits include helping with stress management, calming the mind of anxious thoughts, and activating the parasympathetic nervous system through breathwork. By restoring harmony in the mind and body, going from feeling frazzled and stressed to calm and collected, you can create an environment in your body that is naturally healing and supportive to your wellness journey.

KEY TAKEAWAYS

- Cardio exercises have wonderful heart-health benefits and promote better circulation, higher energy levels, and mood-boosting chemicals in the brain.

- Strength training promotes lean muscle mass, which supports a healthy metabolism.

- Yoga increases strength, balance, and flexibility in addition to calming the mind and nervous system.

- Qigong and tai chi focus on moving qi energy throughout the body to balance the organs and nervous system.

- There are countless movement classes online, so you can find exercise that is right for you.

PRACTICES TO TRY

- Look up community yoga classes near you. You can often try a class for free to see whether the instructor and style are a good fit.

- Many fitness studios and boutiques offer online streaming workout classes you can take in the comfort of your own home.

- Search for different workout classes on YouTube, such as body weight exercises, HIIT exercises, and yoga. YouTube is the greatest free database of workout videos, and if you find a teacher you like, you can subscribe to their channel.

- If you are interested in tai chi or qigong, look for books or classes that go into more details of this beautiful art form. Even though the movements are slow and steady, they can still help your muscles feel the burn and relax your mind.

Pillar 4: Support Healing

Let's talk about how to support your body when you need deep healing. Although the dietary and exercise advice mentioned in the previous pillars may be enough to take you to a new level of vitality, there are also additional techniques to support you, particularly when you're working with a chronic condition or prolonged illness. Here we'll explore techniques from traditional and alternative medicine that can support you in deep healing.

Some of these forms of healing may sound far-fetched and new to you, so I invite you to explore this section with an open mind and curiosity.

ENERGY WORK

Energy healing is a serene holistic modality that has been used for centuries and is starting to gain mainstream popularity. This form of healing helps bring harmony back to the soul, body, and mind by improving the flow of the body's energy system. Energy healing practitioners believe that when there is blocked energy within the body, it can cause disease and physical symptoms ranging from skin inflammation and digestive issues to more severe physical and mental symptoms. There are many different forms of energy healing used throughout various cultures, but I will be discussing three common forms that you may have already heard of: Reiki, acupuncture, and marma point.

Reiki

Reiki is an energy healing modality originating from Japan. The word *Reiki* itself refers to the universal energy, known as *ki*, that moves through all living and non-living matter. Reiki practitioners learn how to work with healing energy in order to help energy flow in others. It is an ancient lineage that is taught only by those who have been attuned with Reiki energy, and this healing energy is attuned in the practitioner's hands through work with a master trainer. Clients receive Reiki to help with stress and anxiety reduction and physical symptoms like headaches or colds, as well as to help release emotional pain and blockages by releasing the energy associated with certain emotions.

Reiki practitioners work with specific symbols and hand techniques that amplify the energy that is transmitted through them. Many Reiki practitioners work with the chakra system of the body, which are seven energy centers that regulate various physical, emotional, and spiritual experiences. When receiving Reiki healing, you will always be fully clothed and your practitioner will work with your chakra system and any areas of your body where energy may feel stuck. Practitioners will either use very light touch or no touch at all. Many Reiki practitioners, including myself, offer distance Reiki healing sessions, since universal energy is not bound by space or time. In my own Reiki sessions I often infuse crystals, which have healing capabilities and can target specific energetic, spiritual, and emotional blockages.

Acupuncture

Credited with unblocking stagnant energy throughout the body, acupuncture is one of the most common procedures recommended by traditional Chinese medicine. Practitioners insert very small needles in a client's skin at specific energetic points of the body, based on meridians, or energy pathways. Acupuncture is a respected treatment for chronic pain, such as joint pain and lower back pain, and can assist with digestive issues or other physical ailments. Many expecting mothers also receive acupuncture to help with the onset of labor.

There are more than 350 acupuncture points throughout the body, and these points are all connected by energetic pathways that help move energy throughout the body. When the acupuncture needles are inserted in these points, energy flow is stimulated, thus working to free up and move around blocked energy. Acupuncture may be uncomfortable for some, as physical needles are inserted through the skin, although the needles are very small and feel like very tiny pricks.

Marma Point Therapy

Marma therapy is an ancient healing modality originating in India. Marma practitioners refer to the life force energy as *prana*, and focus on applying light pressure to 107 marma points in the body and one point in the mind. These are energy access points to balance the mind, body, and soul. Marma point is believed to have influenced the creation of acupuncture, as it is even more ancient. This form of energy healing is part of Ayurvedic medicine and is used to help balance not only prana but the doshas as well.

People seek out marma point therapy to help with digestive issues or if they have been indulging in not-so-healthy lifestyle practices like eating too many processed foods, experiencing high levels of stress, not sleeping well, not exercising, and so on. Marma works similarly to acupuncture in the sense that it aims to unblock stuck energy throughout the body and bring balance to the physical and mental self. Often marma point therapy is combined with Ayurvedic massage for even better results.

BODYWORK

When you are feeling physically stiff or experiencing muscle or joint pain, bodywork can do wonders to alleviate these ailments. Bodywork practices include massage and chiropractic work on the physical body to restore alignment to your joints and connective tissue. Some bodywork modalities, like massage, are also quite ancient, and there are many different forms of massage available today. The type of bodywork that may be right for you depends on your physical symptoms and your preferred approach. Massage and chiropractic work can still be quite spiritual with the infusion of certain practices.

Massage

Massage is an ancient healing tradition used as a therapy for physical ailments. Massage is given through physical touch, and the massage therapist will work with the muscles and soft tissue of the body to alleviate physical stress. Getting a massage can certainly make you feel more relaxed, but the benefits go way beyond simply feeling chilled out. Additional benefits of massage include improved circulation, improved lymphatic flow, relaxed muscle tension, improved mobility, assistance with injury recovery, and much more.

Some of the most popular forms of massage include deep tissue, Swedish, sports massage, Thai massage, reflexology, and shiatsu, which is a bit similar to acupuncture. When looking for a licensed massage therapist, it's important to research the modality they are trained in so you can find exactly the type of treatment you are looking for.

Chiropractic Work

Chiropractic treatment works on the spine, connective tissue, nervous system, and joints, and is not necessarily as relaxing as getting a massage. Chiropractors adjust the body using very specific movements and sometimes tools to help realign the spine, hips, and other parts of the body. This form of bodywork focuses on fixing physical issues without having to rely on surgery or drugs, and a lot of people seek out chiropractic work as a preventive means as well as for managing joint or bone-alignment issues. It's also beneficial for nerve flow through the spinal column, supporting the transmission of hormones, as well as blood and nerve energy through the brain and body.

Often an injury to the back or neck can compromise this free flow of nerve signals through the spinal cord, leading to other health issues down the road.

Naturopathic Medicine

Naturopathic medicine is a health care system that focuses on preventive care, self-care, and the body's innate healing abilities. This field focuses on harnessing and supporting that healing power through natural means before or instead of relying on pharmaceuticals or surgeries. Naturopathic doctors, much like primary care doctors in Western medicine, attend a four-year naturopathic medical school, receive training in a clinical setting, and are able to work with individuals of all ages. Naturopathic doctors also go through all the basic science courses and curriculum as medical doctors (though they are not typically certified medical doctors), and they use these sciences when diagnosing a patient. However, naturopathic doctors also study many different holistic approaches, and their approach to wellness and natural healing focuses on diagnosing the root cause of a disease, with treatments blending various modalities such as homeopathy, nutrition, complementary medicine, conventional medicine, and even spirituality.

There are many benefits to working with a naturopathic doctor if you are more inclined toward natural healing. Naturopathic doctors focus on the root causes of a symptom or illness rather than primarily treating symptoms. Naturopathic doctors also guide patients to learn how to continually care for themselves and can help create preventive wellness plans to maintain optimal health.

Home Remedies

One of the most useful aspects of holistic wellness is the use of home remedies and homeopathy. There are home remedies for just about every symptom, ailment, or emotional or physical aspect of yourself that you want to give some extra loving care to. You can use natural remedies to boost your energy and add them to your beauty routines, and they can have important functions like bolstering your immune system and creating better sleep hygiene.

Daily Practices to Boost Immunity

Practice meditation and yoga. When you are constantly stressed out and pumping cortisol through your veins, you are suppressing your immune response. It's important to manage stress through daily activities such as meditation or yoga to help activate your parasympathetic nervous system, which helps your immune system work optimally.

Consciously hydrate. Consuming enough fluids in the form of water or tea can help break up mucus and flush out toxins or pathogens.

Take steam baths or regular sauna immersions. Studies show that going in a sauna can help fend off respiratory illnesses or diseases. It also has many other benefits, like improved circulation and water weight regulation.

Get out in the sun. When you can get outside once a day, you are infusing your body with the best source of vitamin D, which helps support your immune system and fight off pathogens that enter your body.

Herbs and Supplements

Elderberry. Research shows this berry can shorten the length of a flu or cold, and it is high in nutrients like vitamin A, beta-carotene (a wonderful antioxidant to support overall health), and vitamin C. It is most commonly consumed in liquid form and has a pleasant sweet taste.

Echinacea. This herb works to bolster the immune system and fend off illnesses, and it has been shown to reduce symptoms from the cold and flu. You can take echinacea in capsule form as a daily supplement or when you feel that a cold is about to come on.

Garlic supplements (or eating raw garlic). Did you know that adding garlic to your routine could support your immunity? Studies show that taking garlic supplements can reduce symptoms of a cold and can even prevent it in the first place.

Astragalus. This herb has been used widely in traditional Chinese medicine and is considered an "adaptogen," which refers to a group of herbs that work to regulate the body's stress response. Astragalus can also help fend off viruses or pathogens that enter the body, and it is commonly included as a powder supplement in smoothies.

Lifestyle Tips

Managing your alcohol intake. Doing so is extremely important in order to keep your immune system strong. When you consume alcohol in excess, it suppresses your immune system, which makes you very susceptible to contracting a virus.

Limiting sugar. Easing off the sugar is important, as it helps your body work better to recover from injury or illness if you do find yourself under the weather.

Regularly consuming foods high in vitamin C and zinc. These are two nutrients that are crucial for maintaining a healthy immune system. Vitamin C can be found in citrus fruits, broccoli, sweet peppers, and papaya. It's important to consume sources of vitamin C every day, as the body does not make it on its own. Zinc can be found in food sources like oysters, lamb, legumes, and whole grains.

Essential Oils

Support immunity with peppermint, orange, cinnamon, and tea tree, as well as eucalyptus, which is great for respiratory health.

Daily Practices to Boost Energy

Acupressure for energy. Acupressure works like acupuncture but without needles. There is a pressure point right between your thumb and index finger known as the "Valley of Harmony," which is the fleshy area of your palm. When you gently press this area with your thumb and pointer finger from the other hand and massage it a bit, it can help perk you up.

Hydrotherapy. All you do is stand under hot water for a few minutes, then transition to cold, and I mean *cold*, water for as long as you can bear it. Repeat this three or four times and notice how you feel both physically and mentally.

Tap your thymus with EFT. Similar to acupressure, Emotional Freedom Technique (EFT) is a natural method for supporting the nervous system. Your thymus is right in the middle of your chest, directly below your collarbone, and when you tap it gently 15 to 20 times, it can clear your mind and boost your energy.

Herbs and Supplements

Ginseng. The two most popular forms of ginseng to take for mental clarity and energy are American ginseng and Asian ginseng. Ginseng acts as a natural stimulant and can aid with concentration or general feelings of fatigue. It's a natural stimulant, so it's important not to take it too late in the day, which can result in insomnia or a later-than-normal bedtime.

Cordyceps. Cordyceps is a mushroom that is used for its energizing properties. It works on a cellular level to improve continual energy levels throughout the day. Cordyceps can be taken in capsule form, but there are also botanical energy drinks that include this mushroom.

Rhodiola. Another herb from the adaptogen family that not only helps with energy, but also assists with how your body responds to stress. It works by reducing cortisol, the stress hormone that increases whenever you feel frazzled.

Green tea or matcha. These teas are most likely in your pantry already. Green tea and matcha will give you a caffeine boost without the jitters that coffee does. I love matcha, specifically, because it is green tea leaves ground up as a whole and consumed in your tea, whereas green tea just infuses the properties from its leaves. Green tea and matcha also provide amino acids and antioxidants that further support your health and boost energy levels.

Lifestyle Tips

Create the right type of morning routine. To get your blood flowing and energy levels up, open your windows and get sunlight in your room to lower your levels of melatonin (the sleepy hormone). Practice some stretches to get your blood flowing, go for a quick walk, and then create a creative morning ritual like journaling, reading from your favorite book for 20 minutes, or doing something that will stimulate your mind (without staring at a phone).

Working out midday. Fatigue often strikes in the afternoon. To fend off the midday slump, work out during or right after lunchtime to boost your energy and your mood.

Essential Oils

Uplifting oils include lemon, peppermint, rosemary, orange, and fir.

Daily Practices to Boost Mood

Yoga. Practicing yoga regularly can help clear your mind and make you feel more calm and content. Even a 10- to 15-minute at-home morning practice can help set the tone for the day ahead.

Journaling. By writing down what you are feeling, you are expressing your emotions and processing them on paper. Journaling can help relieve stress and boost your mood when done consistently, and it can even help change your perspective on the matter at hand.

Create sensory rituals. By connecting with your senses, you can redirect anxious thoughts and stress and practice the art of mindfulness all in one. Rituals can include listening to the wind through the trees outside, appreciating the feel of sun on your skin, and getting cozy under a weighted blanket while sipping your favorite beverage and savoring the flavor.

Herbs and Supplements

Omega-3. Research shows this healthy fat can help with depression, including postpartum. You can take omega-3 in supplement form or find it in foods like fatty fish, walnuts, and chia seeds.

Saint-John's-wort. Studies have shown the benefits of this herb in treating depression, and it is also safe to take as a postpartum mother (although it's still very important to get the go-ahead from your doctor before trying any new supplement). It will take some time for the herb to build up in the body in order to create an effect, so give it a few weeks to start working.

Probiotics. Probiotics have been shown to support not only mood but brain health, too. This is because of what is known as the brain-gut axis, where your gut and brain are connected via your nervous system.

Lifestyle Tips

Prioritize alone time. In modern society, it seems like alone time can be fleeting, especially for those who have families or live with roommates. It's extremely important to have time for yourself each day so that you can sit with your own thoughts, do activities you enjoy, and take a break from everyday responsibilities.

Be social. You've already learned about the importance of human connections. By maintaining healthy relationships and connecting with others, you will be supporting your emotional and mental health.

Keep your space tidy. When your home is clear of clutter, your mind will feel clear as well. Next time you feel frazzled, try organizing a drawer in your home or straightening up your bedroom. Notice the immediate difference in your mood!

Essential Oils

Studies have shown that certain essential oils, like lavender, may have antidepressant effects. Clary sage, jasmine, patchouli, ylang ylang, and chamomile all can have a grounding effect on the mind, and can also help downregulate your nervous system when inhaled.

Daily Practices for Weight Management

Take at least 10,000 steps a day. Doing so ensures that you are moving throughout the day and can also increase your energy levels by getting your circulation moving.

Chew slowly. Did you know that being mindful about how you chew can help with weight management? Studies show that chewing slowly can help prevent overeating and can stimulate weight-management hormones.

Experiment with meal prepping. When you take the time one day a week to make parts of meals or whole meals ahead of time, you are saving yourself time during the remainder of the week *and* reducing the likelihood you'll give into cravings, because you'll already have something ready to eat in the fridge.

Herbs and Supplements

Black pepper. You most likely already have this common spice in your pantry. Black pepper contains a compound that has been linked to the inhibition of fat cell formation.

Cayenne pepper. This spicy pepper is commonly used in cooking to add flavor and heat. Research shows that consuming cayenne pepper can increase metabolism throughout the day (meaning you'll burn more calories).

Apple cider vinegar. This vinegar is so popular, it even comes in supplement pill form. When consumed in small quantities, apple cider vinegar can help balance insulin levels, which helps reduce cravings. It can help ease digestive upsets, too.

Ginger. Ginger not only helps regulate weight management, but it can also help with many digestive troubles like nausea, bloating, and indigestion. You can add ginger to your smoothies, soups, and stir-fries and even enjoy it as a crystalized chew.

Lifestyle Tips

Focus on protein for the first meal of your day. When you have a protein-packed meal as your first meal of the day, it reduces cravings for the remainder of the day, helps balance your hunger hormones, and keeps your blood sugar stable so that you don't get a surge of energy and then crash and crave.

Practice mindful eating. Mindful eating means not multitasking when you're eating. When you are present during your eating experience, you are fully aware of the flavors, texture, and experience of your meal. This practice will help you realize when you are full and can help you feel more satisfied with your meals.

Sleep longer. When you are sleep deprived, your appetite increases and cravings can run amok. By getting the right amount of sleep and waking up feeling refreshed, you won't need to look for additional sources of fuel to keep going (aka an overabundance of food).

Essential Oils

Certain essential oils, like grapefruit, have been shown to potentially help the body effectively break down fat as well as reduce cravings. Cinnamon essential oil can also help reduce sugar cravings.

Daily Practices for Sleep

Create a tranquil evening routine. Wind down in the evening by turning all devices off an hour before bed. Infuse your room with calming scents, and get any thoughts out of your head by writing down your to-do list for the next day. Practicing breathwork and meditation before bed can help calm the mind.

Epsom salt bath. Magnesium is the number-one property in Epsom salts, and when the magnesium is absorbed into your system via your skin, it can relieve muscle soreness, relax the nervous system, and help promote better sleep.

Evening self-massage. Self-massage is a lovely self-care practice you can incorporate into your evening routine, and it can help reduce pain and stressful thoughts. It has also been shown to help people who've been experiencing insomnia.

Herbs and Supplements

Magnesium. If you aren't a fan of taking Epsom salt baths, you can still supplement with magnesium to get the same benefits to promote restful sleep and prevent insomnia.

Glycine. This amino acid helps regulate the nervous system and works to lower your body temperature at bedtime in order to prevent restless sleep. Unlike some other sleep aids, such as melatonin, glycine is not believed to induce a groggy aftereffect the next morning.

Valerian root. This root originated in Europe and Asia and is gaining popularity as a supplement in the United States. It has been used to treat symptoms of anxiety, and it is also a common herbal sleep aid.

Lifestyle Tips

Create a sanctuary in your room. Make sure your bedroom creates an inviting, calming energy. Install blackout curtains to keep the room dark, and keep it tidy and free of clutter.

Avoid late-night munching. When you eat later in the evening, especially carbohydrates or fatty foods, it can disrupt your sleep because your digestive system will have to continue working throughout the night. The earlier you eat dinner, the more of a break you will give your digestive system so it can rest and repair.

Essential Oils

One of the best uses for essential oils is for sleep assistance. Many essential oils are used to promote rest and relaxation, which will help you sleep better. Lavender essential oil is the most common scent to promote sleep, and frankincense, chamomile, and vanilla are also great for this purpose. Set a diffuser next to your bed so you can take in the scents as you're falling asleep. (Essential oils are very potent, so it's important never to ingest them, and they should touch your skin only if they've been heavily diluted with water.)

KEY TAKEAWAYS

- Supportive healing can be a wonderful, holistic approach to incorporate in your self-care practice, in addition to treatment from a medical doctor.

- Reiki, acupuncture, and marma point therapy work with the energy centers of the physical body to break up stagnant energy and create free-flowing movement of energy throughout the body.

- Massage and chiropractic work focus on realigning and adjusting the physical body to manage pain and treat ailments.

- Naturopathic medicine is an alternative medical approach that focuses on natural, holistic alternatives to managing illness.

- There are numerous home remedies you can incorporate into your routine to help boost your energy, immune system, and mood and to improve sleep.

PRACTICES TO TRY

- Find a credentialed energy work healer in your area or one who is able to work remotely.

- Find a spa that offers holistic services like shiatsu massage, acupuncture, or aromatherapy massage to experience the wonderful benefits of bodywork.

- Chiropractic work can support more than an aching back or neck. This modality could help you with sleep and digestive issues as well as a weakened immune system and other challenges.

- If you are looking for alternative ways to manage issues like infertility, hormone imbalance, or autoimmunity, visit a naturopathic doctor to develop a holistic treatment plan.

- Consider self-healing through home remedies and watch the shift in your sleep, moods, and duration of colds and flus.

- If you are new to essential oils, find a starter pack and have fun incorporating different scents or blends into your day.

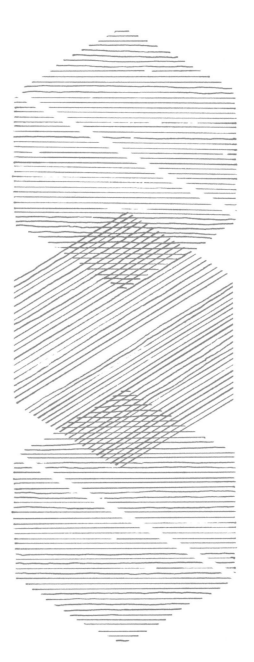

Chapter 4

DESIGN A SELF-CARE ROUTINE FOR PHYSICAL WELLNESS

////////////////////////////////////

There was quite a bit of information packed into part 2! You learned how to self-assess your body type with Ayurveda to get a new perspective on what holistic practices can support your unique body. You also learned about various forms of exercises in order to get an idea of what can work best for your body and current goals. You learned about the dietary practices and lifestyles of those who live in the Blue Zones, and the various nutrient-dense superfoods that can support your body from a cellular level.

Finally, you learned about different holistic approaches to healing the physical body. With all this new knowledge, you will be able to create an encompassing plan to support your physical body in order to continue living a revitalized and vibrant life! Answer the following guided self-inquiry questions to help shape your unique action plan.

GUIDED SELF-INQUIRY

» What is my current morning routine? How can I make it more conducive to promoting sustainable energy throughout the day?

» What are my daily eating habits like? What can I improve about my eating habits? How could I add more fresh plants and whole grains?

» What three types of movements can I start incorporating into my weekly routine? What days can I add these workouts into my schedule?

» What is my current evening routine? How can I make it more conducive to promoting deep and restorative sleep?

» How would I rate the quality of my sleep from 1 to 10? What natural remedies or wellness practices can I incorporate into my day to help improve my sleep?

» What are 10 healthy foods that I enjoy and can incorporate more of into my diet?

» What body type resonates with me, and what daily practices based on my Ayurvedic body type can I start incorporating into my routine?

» What can I do to start experimenting with how energy moves throughout my body to better understand how I can add energy healing into my unique wellness program?

» Do I have any physical pain in my body that can be addressed and worked on through bodywork like massage or chiropractic? If so, where is this pain, and are there additional methods to relieve this symptom?

» What are my favorite scents that make me feel energized, inspired, and calm? How can I incorporate them throughout my day?

SET YOUR INTENTION

As you answer your self-inquiry questions about your physical health, what type of intention comes to the forefront of your mind? Think of your physical self from a holistic standpoint: Are you generally tired? Do you feel bloated and uncomfortable regularly? Do you wish you felt more balanced? See if you are experiencing any particular type of pain point, and set your intention to work through and resolve this pain point from all that you've learned in this pillar.

CREATE YOUR ACTION PLAN

Now that you have your intention set and a good assessment of your physical health, it's time to create your action plan. This action plan will incorporate movements and specific workouts you can start adding to your week based on your current fitness level and how you'd like to feel.

This action plan can also incorporate eating shifts you can make. Try jotting down what you eat for two weeks to see if there are any particular patterns or cravings you are experiencing. From this list, see which "hero foods" you can add more of into your diet. You can also start experimenting with different forms of supportive healing by booking yourself a massage, acupuncture, or energy healing session to see which one works for you.

Here are some prompts to get you started. As a reminder, you can also visit the Practices to Try sections at the end of each pillar. These sections may provide some inspiration for what you'd like to incorporate into your action plan.

A WELLNESS PLAN FOR MY BODY

Actions I will take to support my body:

Action 1:
Action 2:
Action 3:
Three foods I can add to my diet this week:
Three days I will add more movement this week:
My new morning routine:
My new evening routine:

MY IDEAL DAILY SCHEDULE

Your ideal daily schedule should include actionable items that meet your goals for your physical health. This could be creating your own meal plan for each day of the week and also scheduling the days that you will add movement or exercise.

5:00 am	
6:00 am	
7:00 am	
8:00 am	
9:00 am	
10:00 am	
11:00 am	
12:00 pm	
1:00 pm	
2:00 pm	
3:00 pm	
4:00 pm	
5:00 pm	
6:00 pm	
7:00 pm	
8:00 pm	
9:00 pm	
10:00 pm	

PART 3
SPIRIT

Do you believe you have a connection to something greater than life on earth? This could be your religious roots, your awareness of a higher divine being, or a sense that everyone and everything are connected. This is your spiritual belief. In this third and final part, Spirit, we will explore different belief systems, rituals, and thought-provoking questions so you can cultivate a deeper understanding of your spirituality and how you can further connect (or create a connection) with your spirit or soul.

Spiritual well-being is the third part of living a balanced, holistic, and rich life. It is truly unique to each and every one of us, just as everything within mind-body wellness is. The four pillars in part 3 will help you reflect on questions about your soul's purpose, consider how you are spending your time, and determine whether you're pursuing your passions and destiny and actively searching for inspiration to live a fulfilling holistic lifestyle.

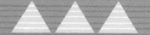

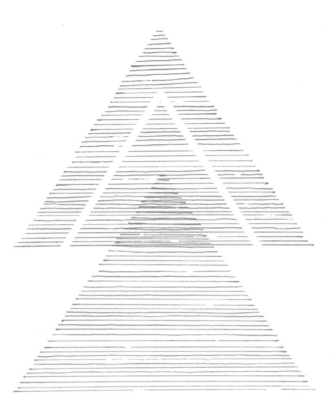
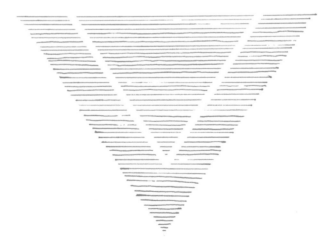

Chapter 5

FOSTERING SPIRITUAL WELLNESS

////////////////////////////////

In this chapter, we'll explore four pillars of spirituality. The first pillar will focus on creating sacred space and time, and will help you learn how to open up some space in your daily life in order to contemplate spiritual matters. The second pillar will unveil the wonder behind your spiritual, mental, and emotional wellness in its connection to nature. The third pillar will help you understand the importance of human connection and how creating meaningful relationships can increase your spirituality. Finally, in the fourth pillar, we will dive into the importance of uncovering your life's passion and destiny in order to work toward something that makes you feel truly alive and free.

Pillar 1: Create Sacred Space and Time

As humans, we are pulled in so many directions. We spend one minute thinking about work, the next minute getting distracted by a notification on our phone, and then we're running off to an important meeting or errand. Because our culture is deeply fixated on always being busy, it can be hard for many of us to carve out time to simply be in the moment, away from our day-to-day responsibilities.

In this pillar, we will first discuss what spirituality means to you as an individual, and then we will explore some ways you can incorporate time for spirituality into your life, no matter how busy you are. I invite you to take a look at your daily and weekly schedules to see whether there are any moments throughout your day or week that can be used for inner work and spiritual growth. How can you make your daily schedule conducive to inner growth, and how much time each day can you dedicate to your inner growth? If you are just beginning, perhaps carve out two or three days a week to work on your spiritual practices, even if it's just for 15 to 20 minutes each day!

DEFINING WHAT INSPIRES YOU SPIRITUALLY

What exactly is spirituality? The concept of spirituality can be very broad and have complex definitions for each of us, but overall it concerns the human spirit or soul. For some, spirituality may include a sense of connection to something larger than your daily, routine existence on Earth. Your personal spirituality could include a belief in one god, a universal benevolent energy, or a divine being or multiple beings, or it could involve a feeling of shared humanity. No matter your definition of spirituality, understanding what uplifts and inspires you can be an important part of cultivating well-being and purpose. A simple way to begin investigating your own spiritual life might be asking yourself what lifts you up and puts you in touch with how meaningful it is to be alive.

So, how do you go about creating the space and time to attend to your inner wellness and growing the spiritual dimension in your life? Here are a few practices that you can start incorporating into your day that can help cultivate a spiritual practice. Before you reflect on what will work for you, take some time to ponder what type of spirituality most resonates with you. It could be your religion, a nonreligious spiritual alignment, or a combination of both.

Prayer and Meditation

A client of mine, Mary, identifies with the Christian religion yet wanted to find ways to incorporate more spiritual practices that helped her increase her connection to God as well as the energy of the universe. She had already established a morning and evening prayer routine, so we worked together to incorporate prayer into a spiritual practice of meditation and visualization. She started her practice with a prayer, spent 10 minutes quieting her mind to meditate, and then spent another 10 minutes practicing visualization techniques, based on her prayers, for what she wanted to attract into her life. With the combination of these practices, she was able to elevate her feelings of joy, passion for life, and determination to live out her purpose by creating a deeper connection to her source.

Visualization

Visualization in itself can be a powerful spiritual practice. It is the application of visualizing in your mind a very specific situation, outcome, or dream you have for your life and imagining it as if it is already happening. This practice is widely used for those who believe in the Law of Attraction—that is, what you think about, you manifest.

Other spiritual practices, which we will discuss in more detail in this chapter, can be connecting with nature, serving and helping others, and finding a community of people who lift you up. Simple acts such as writing down what you're grateful for every day, taking time to reflect on what you believe the meaning of life is, and practicing nonjudgment and compassion toward other humans are small shifts you can start making to bring more spirituality into your life.

CLEARING CLUTTER

What should we do first when we want to create the space and time to bring more spirituality into our homes? Clear out all the clutter. When there is clutter in our homes, our minds and emotions can feel cluttered as well. A cluttered home can make us feel overwhelmed, anxious, and generally stressed out. Our homes should act as our sanctuaries away from everyday stresses, a retreat to relax and contemplate in.

When your home is disorganized, you can become overstimulated and distracted. This is especially problematic if you work from home and are exposed to this type of environment daily. A messy house can send signals to your brain that there is a never-ending to-do list (in addition to your to-do list for other areas of your life), which can leave you feeling like you can never fully relax. This type of mess can trigger anxiety and even suppress productivity and creativity.

There is no doubt, then, that getting your home in order and clearing out the clutter is a necessary first step to evoking inner peace, fulfillment, and focus. Here are a few ways you can clear out your space to welcome in more free-flowing energy and good vibes:

1. Start with one room at a time. Assess any objects in that room that you don't want, don't use, or haven't used in a very long time. If any objects fit this description, donate or toss them!

2. For objects in this room that you do use, establish designated spaces for them. If you need more storage items in order to keep things organized, such as children's toys or books, it is worth the investment so everything in your home can have its own place. I prefer to store items that don't contribute to the decor in closed wicker boxes so the visual stimuli of these objects is gone.

3. Organize your drawers and closets. Go through the practice of tossing or donating items you don't need or use, then organize what's left. You can find inexpensive drawer organizers online to organize all your silverware or junk drawer items, which will make you feel calmer and refreshed.

4. Start small and set your timer for 10 minutes to pick up after yourself at the end of each day. If you have more than 10 minutes to spare, 15 to 20 minutes of daily pickup is even better! By getting into the habit of picking up after yourself, you'll be avoiding unneeded clutter in your home in the first place.

5. Commit to putting objects back in their assigned places after you've used them. This habit is necessary for creating a clutter-free home and will definitely take practice if you don't already do it.

DESIGNING AN ALTAR, MEDITATION, OR QUIET REFLECTION SPACE

Once you've cleared your home of clutter and distractions, it's time to dedicate a space for your spiritual practice! This space should be used only for prayer or meditation, quiet reflection, journaling, and other spirituality practices, and it will be your dedicated sanctuary to create your own unique rituals and practices.

Many folks refer to this space as an altar. It is possible you associate this term with more mystical types of spiritual practices, but this is a commonly used term for any kind of spiritual space, including those deeper holistic practices. It is simply your own sacred space, a dedicated spiritual corner where you can always retreat and focus on your inner growth.

Your altar can become a focal point for moments of quiet reflection, meditation, or reading. An altar is a completely unique and personal tool, and a place to hold objects that remind you of the best in yourself and your life. These objects can be as simple as a small silk cloth and a candle. In some cultures and traditions, people place images of their beloved ancestors on their altars, or images of deities or spiritual teachers who provide inspiration.

Your altar should be in a location that isn't easily disturbed by pets or children. It might be an out-of-the-way spot that helps you slow down for a pause in your day. However, some people like to include a small altar in their kitchens or other busy spaces to serve as a reminder of good things whenever they glance at it. If you live somewhere with nice weather year-round, you could place your altar in a garden or outdoor area. Even creating an altar on your nightstand will work.

What you decide to place on your altar should symbolize what brings you joy and inspiration. The following are some examples of types of items you may choose to include. Use these examples as inspiration to think of items in your home that you can use, or holistic tools you can source.

Sentimental Items

Items that have significant meaning can be placed on an altar to symbolize important people or milestones in your life. Some examples of sentimental items could be a ticket stub from a first date you had with your partner, an item your child crafted for you, or a piece of jewelry handed down from a relative. These items should bring back memories of love, joy, and commemoration when you look at them.

Items That Support Reflection and Contemplation

Whenever I use my meditation altar, I feel inspired to write down new ideas or solutions that come to mind, so I always have a journal and pen stowed away at my altar. You can use a journal to write down what you want to manifest in your life, feelings that need to be expressed, or inspirational thoughts that pop up as you meditate. Other items that can be used for contemplation could be a rosary or mala beads, both of which are strands of beads that are used in prayer and meditation. Angel cards, oracle cards, or tarot cards are also wonderful tools for tapping into your inner guidance. These cards are pulled intuitively, and the messages on each card can give you new insights or perspectives into specific questions you think about or how you can move forward with your day.

Items to Support Your Senses

Did you know that you can tap into all your senses to turn on your parasympathetic nervous system and help your body naturally shift into a meditative state? If you are feeling burned out or overwhelmed, use your altar to tap into your senses and calm racing thoughts, bringing more harmony to your mind and body. Place freshly cut roses on your altar to smell and admire, light candles to gaze at, wrap a shawl or scarf around yourself to feel cozy, or make pleasing sounds using a singing bowl or a bell.

Texts That Inspire You

Your altar can also be used to hold items that help you connect with your faith and reconnect with spiritual teachings. Having meaningful texts on hand—like a collection of sacred poems, the Tao Te Ching, the Bible, the Koran, or the yoga sutras. These texts can support your prayer or contemplation practice. Other religious symbols, like a cross or statues of deities, can also be placed on your altar.

Once you have a space for your altar and your items that will go on it, it is ready to use for your spiritual practice. Here you can practice meditation, prayer, or any ritual you hold close to your heart. You can use your altar whenever you'd like, and just having it there and seeing it throughout the day can trigger a sense of calm in you.

WORKING WITH SYMBOLISM

Making your living space inviting, inspiring, and energizing doesn't just involve keeping it clean and tidy. Working with symbolism is another refreshing way to connect with your home on a deeper level and turn it into a sanctuary that nurtures your soul. If you are at home reading this book right now, I want you to take a look at the room you are in and scan for objects, artwork, or any items that have symbolic meaning to you. Perhaps they elicit specific emotions and moods that stem from a fond memory or represent a specific person or place.

Examples of symbolism can likely be found all over your home. Perhaps you've gone on many travels and brought home vases or sculptures from every town you've visited. These items represent your love for travel and the places you've been. Family photos are obvious symbols of your family unit and special memories you share. Furniture can also hold symbolism, if it was passed down from your parents or extended family, found in a special boutique, or owned previously by someone you admire. All the items on your bookshelf can symbolize the knowledge you've acquired, as well as your interests and passions. No matter what you see around you, how can you study the objects you own to uncover what they represent?

Feng shui is a holistic practice that works with physical spaces and homes to balance energy and promote harmony and peace. Symbolism is very important in feng shui, as feng shui consultants use specific statues and items that stand for things like wealth, love, family, and health. You can pull some ideas from feng shui by thinking of parts of your life that you want to uplift a bit more and sourcing objects that symbolize these parts of your life. For example, if you want to bring more wealth into your life, what objects remind you of living a luxurious life? It could be furniture, a specific piece of art or home decor, or an accolade you are proud of hung in your office.

No matter what you want to draw into your life, you can make your space support your needs and desires. It's also important to scan your home and replace any items that evoke sad memories or items you simply do not use or appreciate. Every six months or so, I take a day to go from room to room and assess the vibe, checking whether there are any items in there that are broken, can be donated, or just have sad energy behind them. I then take note of the emotions and qualities I want to express in my home and reflect on what objects I can incorporate into each space that will symbolize these specific qualities. It's a practice I love to do, and it's something that can really transform your home into a beautiful, inspiring retreat.

By being selective about what you surround yourself with, you will always be reminding yourself of fond memories, people you love, and ideas that inspire you!

PRACTICING PRAYERS, BLESSINGS, OR AFFIRMATIONS

Do you know the power of affirmations and prayers? When you shift your self-talk to that of positive encouragement, self-love, and reassurance, you are quite literally training your brain to believe and act out these thoughts. Practicing prayers, blessings, and affirmations helps fend off negative thoughts and possible self-sabotage, because you are repeating these positive messages to the point that you start to embody your thoughts, which leads to positive growth and change.

Affirmations are thoughts or statements you can say aloud that give you encouragement, confidence, or whatever positive mood you are seeking to embody. Positive affirmations, when used consistently, work by shifting your thinking patterns and getting you unstuck from the negative. They are a great practice when you are cultivating a growth mindset, and studies show that they can boost problem-solving skills and may improve confidence and combat depression. Affirmations can be incorporated into your morning or evening routine, or whenever you feel like you need to shift your self-talk.

Prayers and blessings are two other wonderful ways to shift your mindset and connect with your divine source, regardless of whether you are religious. Your prayers and/or blessings will be unique to your individual traditions, beliefs, and background. Prayers are usually conversations, requests for guidance, or contemplations you have directly with your divine source. Prayers can be made to your god or gods, the universe, or whatever spiritual source you connect with. Blessings, on the other hand, are a means to express gratitude for all that our divine source has given us. Examples of blessings are giving thanks before your meal, delivering words during baptisms or weddings, or wishing someone well. Prayers and blessings can be used at any time of the day but can be especially helpful before you go to bed as you reflect on the day's activities.

KEY TAKEAWAYS

◆ Spiritual wellness is a highly individual practice and looks different for everyone.

◆ Consider making your home a better sanctuary by clearing clutter, simplifying the space to promote calm.

◆ Having a designated spiritual space, or altar, gives you a place of retreat that symbolizes the importance of self-care in your life.

◆ Your home should be full of items that symbolize love, freedom, joy, creativity, and productivity.

◆ Prayers, blessings, and affirmations can shift your mindset, connecting you with your deeper self or your source of wisdom.

PRACTICES TO TRY

◆ Add time to your schedule to check in with your spirit, asking yourself what has supported and inspired you in recent days.

◆ Before you go to bed, take some time to meditate, pray, or practice visualization for five to 10 minutes to start creating this habit.

◆ Dedicate one day per week to start clearing clutter in your home, focusing on one room at a time. It's amazing how much progress you can make in just four weeks!

◆ Find a space in your home for your altar, and think of any objects you can gather that you already have on hand to use for this new soulful practice.

Pillar 2: Align with Nature

Have you noticed that when you visit a beach or park you begin to relax? In nature, you tend to take in deep, invigorating breaths, and your mind feels at ease. Because we are creatures of the earth, and our ancient ancestors lived on the land, our connection with nature is deeply ingrained. Spending time in nature nurtures the spirit, brings us comfort, and can spark inspiration when we need it most.

In this pillar, you will learn various ways you can create a stronger connection to the earth through holistic lifestyle practices. First, we'll explore why nature can be such a strong spiritual support for us. Then we'll take a look at a few ways you can increase this bond, including aligning with the sun and moon cycles, connecting directly with the earth through "grounding" or "earthing," and practicing forest bathing to bring balance to your entire being.

UNDERSTANDING OUR DEPENDENCE ON NATURE

Our relationship with nature is a sacred and visceral connection, passed down since the days of our earliest ancestors. Perhaps this is why spending time on the beach or in the forest—or even at a park—seems to create a shift within us, calming our spirits and reinvigorating our minds. Our senses come alive, igniting feelings of renewal and peace, and the connection to our inner guidance may feel stronger.

As humans, we are innately tied to our environment. Our ancestors lived their entire lives connected to and dependent upon the land around them. Their knowledge of the terrain, including its prospects for food and resources as well as danger, made them highly sensitive to the natural world. They relied on the seasons, weather patterns, the migrations of wild animals, the cycle of planting and harvest, and many other rhythms of nature. In modern life, we still depend greatly on the natural world from the foods we eat to the air we breathe. We know intuitively that we are connected to our environment in more ways than one.

There is a growing body of research that explores how being immersed in nature helps us heal on a deep level. The field of ecopsychology is dedicated to researching our relationship with nature, which is examined through psychological and ecological theories. By better understanding the emotional ties we have with our natural environment, some medical professionals are enriching therapeutic practices by incorporating immersive nature-based experiences.

All types of health systems, from ancient holistic practices to modern Western medicine, have touted the benefits of connecting with nature. In Ayurveda, for example, living in rhythm with nature every day is considered the foundation of health. From a traditional medical standpoint, the evidence and research behind this relationship is clear. Countless studies have uncovered the profound benefits to be gained from spending more time outdoors, including regulating stress, calming the nervous system, lowering blood pressure, and bolstering the immune system. Even a daily short walk outside can make us feel calmer, more connected, and happier.

Unfortunately, the rise in technology seems to keep us indoors longer and pull us away from the natural world. Think about your daily routine. Do you consistently pause throughout your day to listen to the birds outside? How often do you intentionally go to a park to just be in the moment and daydream? Do you often pause to watch the clouds go by, or gaze at the trees waving rhythmically in the wind? If not, there are numerous ways you can rekindle your relationship with nature. Let's take a deeper look at these methods.

LIVING BY SUN AND MOON CYCLES

Have you ever noticed that when you go to bed and wake up around the same time consistently, your energy levels seem a bit more stable? Just as we crave patterns throughout our days when it comes to work or how we go about our morning routine, our body craves its own routine, called the circadian rhythm.

The circadian rhythm is our body's 24-hour cycle. This unique system of hormonal and enzymatic fluctuations is responsible for when we wake up for the day, turn in for bed, and even need to eat. It's a quite predictable biological pattern, and it thrives on consistent routine.

Circadian rhythm is ruled by a part of the brain that takes in signals from the environment around us. These cues consist mainly of temperature and sunlight fluctuations, which signal the brain to release hormones that make us feel drowsy, like melatonin, or that help us wake up, like cortisol. When the sun rises and our eyes can sense this change in light, the brain sends signals to our body that it's time to rise and shine. The same goes for when it gets dark outside; our eyes, adjusting to the lack of light, send another signal to our brain that in turn triggers us to feel tired.

The circadian rhythm also governs digestion as well as women's reproductive cycles, not just when we feel tired or awake.

When we throw off our circadian rhythm by traveling or looking at blue light from screens at night, for example, we are disrupting the production of melatonin, which is the hormone that helps us drift to sleep. In addition to affecting quality of sleep, an out-of-whack circadian rhythm can also negatively impact our mood by exacerbating symptoms of anxiety and depression. This is because sleep disruption affects our cortisol levels, and this imbalance can contribute to these conditions. When we don't get proper sleep, we are also not allowing our bodies the time to fully recover, repair, digest, and detox, which in the short term can lead to difficulty concentrating and staying alert the next day, but can also lead to major health problems down the line.

So, how can we create a daily routine that supports our circadian rhythm? Here are some techniques to consider incorporating:

- Keep a consistent bedtime and set your wake-up alarm for the same time each day.

- Open up your blinds right away when you wake up in the morning to get exposure to natural light as soon as possible.

- Spend time outdoors as often as possible throughout the day to expose yourself to the natural cycle of sunlight.

- Try to limit screen time before bed, and keep TVs and other electronics out of your bedroom. Taking a break in the evening will help your body reset and return to its natural patterns.

- Manage your stress throughout the day by keeping active and practicing mindful stress-coping practices like meditation.

- Make dinner your lightest meal so your digestion doesn't have to work overtime at night.

EARTHING

If you've ever enjoyed the fresh feeling of grass beneath your feet at the park or the sand between your toes on a visit to the beach, you've already experienced the practice known as "earthing" or "grounding." It's a simple yet powerful way to support your emotional and spiritual benefits.

And there is science behind the practice. There are naturally occurring electrical charges within our bodies, made up of what are known as free radicals, which are oxygen molecules that are reactive or unstable and create an electrical charge. When you hear about inflammation in the body, it is usually a result of these free radicals damaging our other healthy cells. Eating antioxidant-rich foods is one way to fend off these free radicals. However, earthing may be another way to keep them at bay and lower inflammation.

The earth has an abundance of free electrons, which means it can actually "ground" the free radicals in our bodies by bonding with these unstable molecules, thus reducing inflammation and other health issues in the body. Multiple studies support the effects of grounding on our physical bodies and even its capability for wound healing. Grounding can also improve the quality of your sleep, reduce chronic pain, and help with muscle recovery. So how do you practice earthing? It is actually quite simple, and it only requires being barefoot.

Wearing shoes insulates our feet from the electrical charge of the earth. To practice earthing, you simply need to find a grassy or sandy area, slip off your shoes and socks, and place your hands and feet on the earth. You can also lie down, walk around barefoot for a bit, or simply sit on the ground with your soles on the earth for about 30 minutes. If outdoor access is tricky, some companies now sell grounding mats and products you can stand on to achieve this same benefit.

FOREST BATHING

Even though it sounds like a strange hygiene practice, you don't actually *bathe* in a forest. Forest bathing is simply the practice of spending time out in a beautiful environment, free of skyscrapers and architecture. By immersing yourself in a natural setting and intentionally taking in everything around you, by walking through a forest or lying in a meadow, you are practicing the art of forest bathing. This practice emphasizes the use of your five physical senses, teaching that it's through our senses that we are really able to create this beautiful connection with the earth.

Origins

The concept of forest bathing was born in the 1980s in Japan. The practice originated as a way to deal with the mental and spiritual drain that came from technology overload and living in a densely populated urban setting, like in that country's largest cities. Research on this practice started picking up steam about 10 years later to support the already intuitive benefits of spending time in nature.

Some studies of forest bathing found that the practice lowered blood pressure, decreased levels of the stress hormone cortisol, triggered the parasympathetic nervous system (which is responsible for helping us feel calm), and decreased feelings of depression.

A Simple Forest Bathing Practice

Leave your phone at home or in your car and venture out to a secluded park or uncrowded spot on a nearby beach where you have the space to wander and explore as you wish. Take a slow, peaceful stroll through a forest or wade into the shallow depths of an ocean or lake. Gaze at the sunrise or sunset or simply watch clouds go by.

Wherever your forest bathing spot is, take a few breaths to connect yourself to the moment and open up each of your senses to your surroundings, one by one. Fully take in each smell, each breath, each sound, and each blow of the wind or grain of sand. Really spend this time connecting to your senses.

Let your thoughts start to slow and wander while you appreciate the beauty around you. Begin by noticing all the fragrances, from freshly cut grass to water misting off sidewalks in your local park. Then listen for birds calling, leaves rustling, or water flowing. Move through your senses in this way one by one to appreciate the sensations of the moment. Let go of worries and stay with this practice as long as it feels comfortable.

KEY TAKEAWAYS

- ◆ Our relationship with nature has ancient roots, as our ancestors lived and thrived on the land.

- ◆ Ecopsychology emphasizes therapeutic techniques that help increase our bond with nature in order to feel calm, connected, and joyful.

- ◆ Our bodies crave a consistent sleep/wake routine based on the sun and moon cycles, called the circadian rhythm. Following this rhythm helps us feel alert, energized, and balanced throughout the day.

- Physically connecting with nature through earthing or grounding has benefits beyond making us feel calm and can actually heal our bodies by decreasing inflammation.

- Forest bathing, or spending time in an area that is completely natural, has both physical and mental health benefits.

PRACTICES TO TRY

- Add a walk around your neighborhood to your morning routine by finding a path that leads you to a local park or an area graced by the natural environment.

- Invite nature into your home by bringing in houseplants and greenery.

- Practice forest bathing by finding a quiet spot out in a park or in a forest preserve and let your senses guide your experience.

- Get outside barefoot as much as you can to practice earthing, aligning your body with the healthy electrical energy of the earth.

- Connect with your circadian rhythm by waking earlier with the sun and winding down at dusk to see what bedtime feels good to you.

Pillar 3: Find Your People

Sociological research conducted all over the world, including in the Blue Zones, shows the importance of building healthy relationships in order to support a long and healthy life. When you are involved with your community, building stronger bonds with your family, and nurturing relationships with your friends, you are supporting your emotional and mental well-being, which can literally add years to your life.

In this pillar, we will explore the importance of our closest circle of loved ones and suggest ways to build meaningful relationships with those we care about. We'll discuss community activities, groups, and events to explore for a robust social life. When we nurture and grow the relationships we have, we cultivate a sense of belonging, our innate need for human connection, and our ability to practice more empathy and compassion toward others.

FOSTERING FAMILY TIES

Your family bond can be your constant in a world of uncertainty. In modern times, the idea of "family" has evolved and may not be limited to your biological relatives like parents and children but might also include your chosen family of close friends.

For some people, family is who you come home to after a long day to share stories and break bread with. Healthy family relationships provide a deep sense of belonging and support during tough times. Your family can be your source of growth, stability, happiness, and confidence. If you have children, providing a nurturing, loving home can help them feel safe and loved.

It also important to mention that not every family dynamic is uplifting and positive. Although resolving a family conflict and reuniting with an estranged relative can be healing, it is not always possible. Sometimes it's wise to save your energy for the healthier, more meaningful connections in your life rather than struggle with a toxic relationship. It's absolutely okay to prioritize your well-being and set healthy boundaries.

Plenty of studies support the importance of family and its link to better health and wellness. Having strong family ties throughout life gives you a greater sense of purpose, improving emotional and psychological health, which in turn contributes to longer life spans and disease prevention. Studies also show that being happily married is linked to better physical and mental health.

Regardless of whether you live with family members, here are some ideas from various cultures and traditions to help you bond, connect, and spend quality time with the people you love.

Exchanging Family Stories

Making the time to have meaningful conversations with family can nurture relationships and elicit happy nostalgia. Asking elders to share their stories or telling your own children exciting stories from your childhood can bring them comfort, reminding them that we all go through ups and downs and have many feelings over a lifetime. On date nights with your partner, remember to swap stories from your childhoods. There's always more to learn about another human, even if we've lived with them for years.

Create Family Altars

Many cultures celebrate ancestors and loved ones by creating some form of family altar. In Japan, family altars are called *butsudan* and are usually created as a memorial for elders who have passed away. Family members set offerings on these altars—usually objects that had meaning to the deceased loved one. You can create a family altar in your home by choosing a spot for framed photos of your ancestors. As a healing ritual, choose one day a week to set fresh flowers or "offerings" that have meaning between you and the deceased.

Dedicate a Few Days a Week to Family Mealtime

Many studies confirm the importance having dinner together as a family. Sharing meals creates the opportunity to tell stories, spend quality time together, and, if you have kids, show them the stability that comes with eating together as a family.

Care for Animals Together

A beautiful tradition in India is to celebrate the importance of animals by feeding birds and cows during an annual festival. Children grow up learning that all species, especially animals, are interconnected and should be respected and loved. This cultural tradition can be re-created by simply visiting a petting zoo or farm, where you can teach your children the importance of being kind to animals or how to care for them.

Share Your Favorite Pastimes and Games

When you encourage your family to participate in your favorite hobbies, you are bringing your loved ones together to do something you are passionate about. This activity can be anything from cooking meals to trying new creative art projects to playing your favorite games.

BUILDING MEANINGFUL RELATIONSHIPS

Fostering meaningful relationships with those outside your family can bring just as much fulfillment and benefit for your well-being. In today's digital world, it's easy to lose touch with the importance of in-person connection. Digital connections can be engaging, but there's nothing better than quality, in-person time for building great friendships.

There are many ways you can connect with others to cultivate rich relationships, and they all encompass respecting each other, connecting through shared interests or shared experiences, and upholding values together. It's also important to learn how to truly listen to and understand those you care about.

Have you ever gone through phases in your life when you felt completely misunderstood? Maybe throughout your childhood you had periods when you were teased or bullied for being different. If you had anyone in your life at that time who listened to your frustrations and made your voice heard, do you remember how that made you feel? It can be a huge relief when someone recognizes your experiences and lets you express yourself. You can also be this sounding board for others by practicing active listening. Put away your phone, make eye contact, and listen to the other person with full attention. Ask questions and listen with empathy and nonjudgment. Showing your loved ones this respect and care deepens your connection.

Connecting with others through shared interests is another great way to nurture existing relationships as well as start new ones, and it can be quite easy to do, especially as you meet someone for the first time. When you meet a new potential friend, instead of telling them about yourself, ask about their hobbies, their job, their favorite restaurants, or their family.

If you want to strengthen your current relationships, plan special outings around things you both love to do. Some examples could be taking cooking or other classes together, working out or staying active together by going on jogs, or volunteering for a cause you both are passionate about.

You can also connect through shared values by celebrating a holiday or practicing your religious or spiritual rituals together, or taking action together to support a cause that has great meaning to both of you. Doing so can lead to great memories and fulfilling moments that bring you closer together.

CONNECTING WITH YOUR COMMUNITY

Connecting with your community can help contribute to your longevity, mental wellness, and feelings of joy and belonging. Even if you're not necessarily an extrovert, there are still many ways that you can put yourself out there to connect with new friends in your community that won't make you feel uncomfortable.

Studies have shown the importance of community connections, especially during periods of crisis or adversity. One study showed that individuals who had a robust social life lived longer, regardless of socioeconomic status and whether they smoke, drank, or were physically active.

There are many ways to get to know your community. To start, local volunteer opportunities can naturally connect you with others who share your values and beliefs.

You can also search for local groups organized around a specific interest or life event. A birth prep class or new moms group are examples. Other groups are formed around business goals, perhaps tied to a specific industry or field. There are also many book clubs, writing groups, wellness and fitness groups, or others that gather around a particular hobby. One popular website for finding groups or gatherings is Meetup.com, which lists upcoming happenings in your city.

Other ideas include joining an adult sports league or seeking out cultural events, fairs, block parties, town festivals, local art shows, and live musical performances. No matter the activity, there are many ways to gather around shared interests and connect with your community.

KEY TAKEAWAYS

- Social connection is a major contributor to a healthy and happy life.

- Having close ties to family and/or chosen family supports your emotional and physical health.

- Building and strengthening relationships based on shared interests, values, and respect will help foster bonds and longevity.

- There are numerous ways to get to know your community, deepen your sense of belonging, and support others.

PRACTICES TO TRY

- Find gatherings or events through websites like Meetup.com.

- Join a local sports league if you enjoy being active.

- Experiment with adding a new family tradition, or simply eat dinner together more often.

- Carve out a few nights a week to connect with your partner or a close friend.

- Take time to reconnect with a dear friend or family member if you've fallen out of touch.

Pillar 4: Cultivate Purpose

Now that you've explored how to care for your emotional and mental health, it's time to reflect on the future of your life's journey.

Most of us yearn to live life to its fullest potential, pursuing our dreams and working toward our passions. When you truly connect with your authentic self—the parts of you that are not influenced by society or people around you—it becomes much easier to find and follow your calling.

In this final pillar, we'll discuss deepening that connection to the authentic self in order to unveil our deepest desires, passions, and purpose. Much of our discussion so far has led to this point. When you physically feel amazing and know how to care for yourself, you're freer to take risks—and move ahead toward a life of fulfillment.

To dive in, let's start by exploring what has molded your self-knowledge and identity thus far, and how connected you feel now with your truest self.

KNOWING YOURSELF

When you are grounded in your authentic self, you feel connected to your mind, body, and soul. You often feel safe, assured, confident, and whole—and considerably more resilient when turbulence strikes. You understand what supports your emotional health and what triggers you. You've learned how to bring yourself back on track after setbacks and you know how to express yourself freely with others.

As a child, your primary beliefs about yourself were shaped by your caregivers, as was what you learned about life and humanity. These norms and values may still dictate your life decisions and choices, and impact relationships you have with others as well as yourself. But beliefs rooted in family of origin can sometimes be generational and may not always be healthy to you as an individual.

When you ask yourself, "Who am I?" how is the answer influenced by our family or culture of origin? If you're fortunate, you grew up feeling secure in yourself, free to be yourself and deserving of unconditional love. This type of upbringing makes it easier to express your deepest thoughts and identity to the world now. However, many of us were not quite so lucky. What if you didn't feel safe or comfortable fully being yourself as a child?

I also invite you to think about who your guides and helpers were growing up, and who they are now. Who created a space for you to grow and evolve as your truest self, and who may have inhibited your dreams and passions? This is not an invitation to put blame on others, but is instead a moment to be honest about how much freedom you have had to form your own beliefs and choices about yourself and the world around you.

The good news is, there are many ways to repair and heal from limiting beliefs we heard as children. Take a moment to take stock of how you see yourself and how those views formed over time. Reflect on how old beliefs are shaping your present state and potential future. Consider how you may wish to update your own beliefs to support your deepest desires and dreams.

PURSUING YOUR OWN FULFILLMENT

Do you feel that you are living out your dreams, passions, and interests? Do you fully express your ideas, gifts, and talents?

You can live with purpose, no matter the age or time of life. Blue Zones research found that feeling purposeful every morning was a hallmark of people who live long, robust lives. In Costa Rica, home to one of the Blue Zones, people refer to their purpose as their *plan de vida*, the thing that gets them up in the morning. At one point in life, your purpose may be to start your own business or find a life partner. At another moment, what gets us up in the morning may be teaching a grandchild how to bake cookies, watering the garden, or calling on an old friend.

Purpose is an evolving sensibility but is always important. It drives your subconscious thoughts and actions, and make you feel enthused and inspired.

When you can connect with purpose, a spark forms inside you. Because your purpose changes as you grow, you may find yourself questioning your identity in different chapters of your life, which is completely normal. Discovering and rediscovering dreams, goals, and new purposes can be exciting. So make it a practice to check in with yourself and continually investigate what gives you joy, and what plans and ideas seem to light you up.

The easiest way to start uncovering your passions is by asking yourself what you truly love to do and what seems to come naturally to you. You could have multiple talents and many passions—if so, lucky you! How can you create something for the world that combines your talents and interests so you can do something that you love every day?

Understanding your purpose helps keep your life fresh, dynamic, and meaningful. It helps you learn about yourself and end your day feeling like you've lived that day fully.

SHARING YOUR GIFTS FOR THE GOOD OF ALL

A great source of fulfillment can be serving others. What does service mean to you? It could mean getting involved with a local nonprofit, pursuing activism to fight for what you believe is right, or simply remembering to smile as you greet strangers.

Think about how you've felt when you've been able to lift others up. Even small acts of kindness matter, such as holding open a door for someone or offering to help a coworker with a tedious task. There are studies that link helping others with health benefits, such as a longer lifespan and better mental health.

There are many ways you can help others and share your gifts with the world. And it all starts with embodying the mindset of empathy and love. When you live your life from a place of love, you can touch the hearts of many. If you don't know where to start, try visiting websites like VolunteerMatch.org to find local opportunities to give back. Other ways you can serve others are by donating clothes or personal items to local shelters, or attending meetings about social change or improvements for the community.

By helping others, you are sharing your skills and practicing the art of gratitude—and setting an example for others to do the same!

KEY TAKEAWAYS

◆ Knowing our authentic selves, including our dreams and passions, is important to living a life of wellness.

◆ Reflect on how your past experiences and ingrained beliefs shape your sense of self.

◆ Learning what your life's purpose is will help you pursue your goals with more drive, passion, and energy.

◆ Your purpose can be a combination of your natural talents and what you enjoy doing the most.

◆ Serving others is an expression of gratitude—and a powerful wellness practice!

PRACTICES TO TRY

◆ Write down your thoughts on your family and culture of origin, and how they have influenced your beliefs about yourself and the world. It is okay to notice both positive and negative reflections.

◆ Consider any limiting beliefs that may prevent you from taking risks or expressing yourself fully.

◆ Recall those who have inspired and encouraged you.

◆ Contemplate what your ideal day looks like. Where are you, who are you with, and what are you doing?

◆ Reflect on how you most like to express yourself. When do you currently embody these expressions? Which ones deserve more time and attention?

◆ Evaluate new ways to serve and help others, from daily acts of kindness to volunteering.

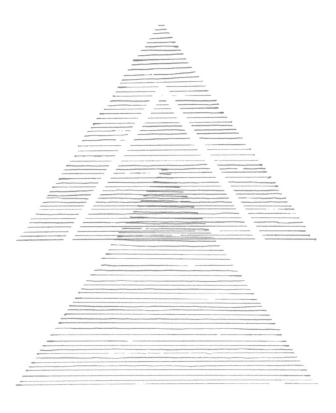
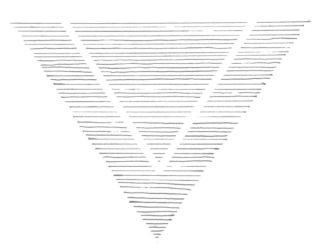

Chapter 6

DESIGN A SELF-CARE ROUTINE FOR SPIRITUAL WELLNESS

////////////////////////////////////

Now that you've been able to explore a few facets of finding connection, inspiration, authenticity, and purpose, it's time to start putting it all together to create a self-care routine for your spiritual wellness!

This routine can incorporate daily spiritual practices pulled from the previous pillars as well as ideas that may not be in this book but you feel drawn to exploring. I also invite you to see how you can carve out time to connect with family and friends on a consistent basis, or find ways you can explore new relationships or connections.

It's very important that you make this routine your own and do what feels right to you. As you reflect on what spirituality means to you and the importance of building connections with others who share similar beliefs and values, your self-care routine may look different than others you have encountered. That's the point!

GUIDED SELF-INQUIRY

» Who am I? What makes up
my identity?

» What are my natural talents?

» In what ways do I enjoy serving or
helping others?

» If I could do anything in the world,
what would it be?

» If I had an entire week to do whatever I wanted each day, what would
my ideal day(s) look like?

» What activities do I participate in
that bring me joy?

» Where or from whom do
I find inspiration?

» What can I start doing on a
regular basis that brings me
a sense of purpose?

» Who do I have in my life to act as
my mentor or life guide?

» What divine source do I identify and
connect with, and how have I been
nurturing this connection thus far?

» What are my top 10 values and
qualities that I want to live out
and express?

» Who in my life lifts me up and supports all my goals and dreams?

SET YOUR INTENTION

Now that you've answered the self-inquiry questions, you may have a greater understanding of what your authentic identity is as well as your spiritual ties and how you
want to express and live out your passions. Now it's time to set an intention for your
spiritual wellness—whether that's getting started with creating a space for spirituality
or religion in your life, strengthening your existing practice, or exploring new ways of
living and being.

CREATE YOUR ACTION PLAN

It's time to put everything you've read into action and create your own unique wellness
plan rooted in spirituality and the intention you've set for yourself! Take advantage
of all the tools you've learned in this book, including the Practices to Try at the end

of each pillar, to make a plan that works for you. It's important that you come back to this plan regularly as you begin your practices, or even make a copy of this plan to place on a wall you frequently walk past. You can do the same for your mental and physical action plans as well. See the following example prompts for inspiration to get started.

A WELLNESS PLAN FOR MY SPIRIT

Actions I will take to support myself spiritually:

Action 1:
Action 2:
Action 3:
What I no longer need:
What I need more of:
Here are my hurdles:
Here are my allies:
On my mind:

MY IDEAL DAILY SCHEDULE

Your ideal daily schedule can be revisited and changed as you move through life. Remember, the plan you make for yourself now is not set in stone forever. I encourage you to change and shift your daily schedule as needed to best fit the evolution of your life.

5:00 am	
6:00 am	
7:00 am	
8:00 am	
9:00 am	
10:00 am	
11:00 am	
12:00 pm	
1:00 pm	
2:00 pm	
3:00 pm	
4:00 pm	
5:00 pm	
6:00 pm	
7:00 pm	
8:00 pm	
9:00 pm	
10:00 pm	

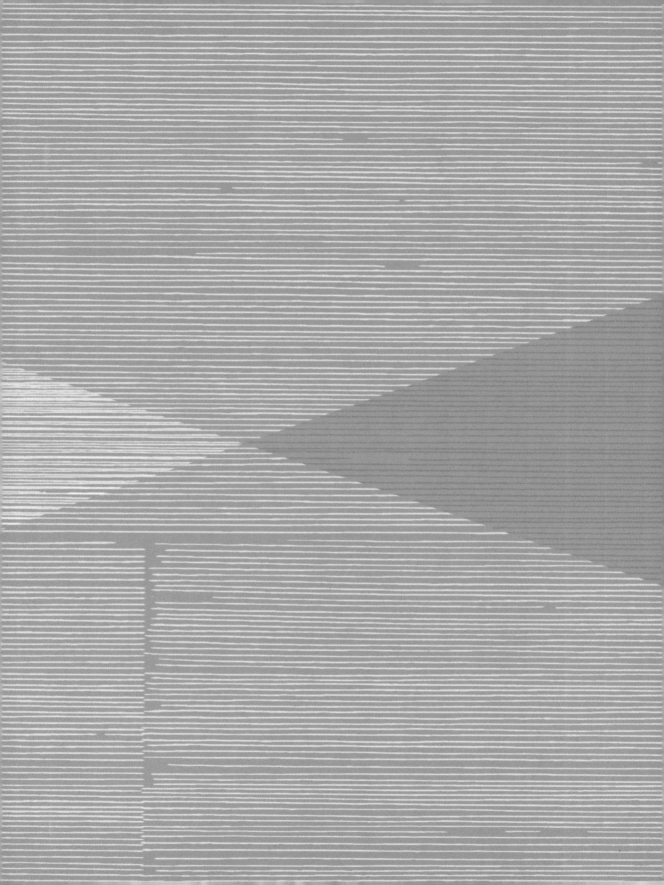

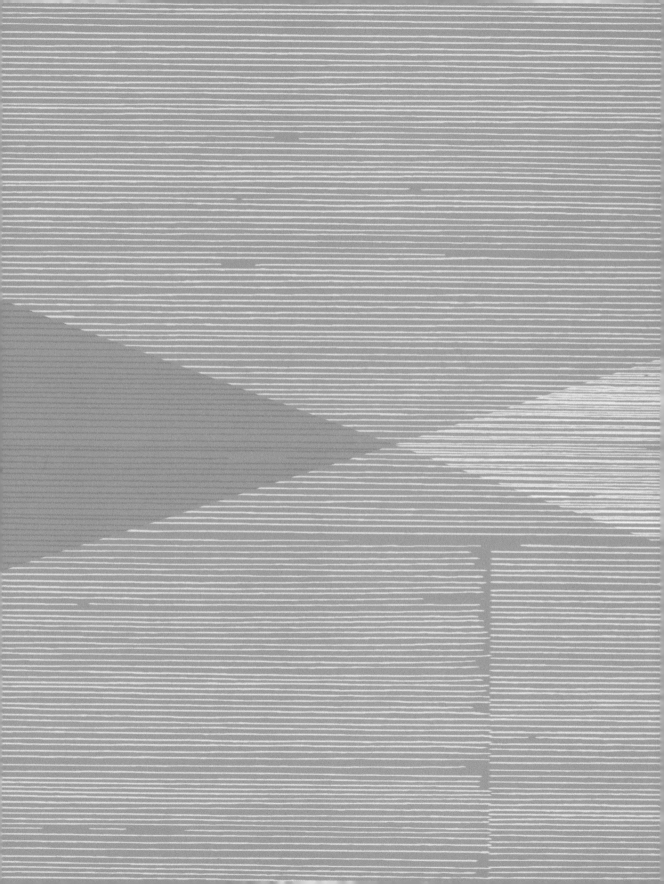

RESOURCES

////////////////////////

Books

The Five-Minute Journal *by Intelligent Change Inc.*
This book is a great starter journal to create your daily gratitude practice. Each day you spend five minutes filling out a page, which helps you reflect on your mental and emotional well-being.

Choosing Gratitude: Your Journey to Joy *by Nancy Leigh Demoss*
This book motivates readers to live with intention and teaches the importance of taking time each day to cultivate gratitude.

The Blue Zones Solution: Eating and Living Like the World's Healthiest People *by Dan Buettner*
If reading about the Blue Zones in this book piqued your interest, you can learn even more from Dan Buettner himself.

Intuitive Eating: A Revolutionary Program That Works *by Elyse Resch and Evelyn Tribole*
This book explores the art of intuitive eating, teaching you to focus on eating healthy without restrictive diets or regimens.

Apps

Gratitude Plus
This app is a great way to incorporate daily gratitude journaling into your routine with a built-in community and other fun features.

Insight Timer
This meditation app has more than 45,000 free meditation and meditative music tracks to choose from to get your meditation practice started immediately.

Adidas Training by Runtastic

This app provides 30 free workouts for every fitness level as well as challenges to participate in and other motivating features to create a consistent workout routine.

Websites

mindful.org

Mindful provides education and free resources on meditation, mindfulness, and conscious living.

mindbodygreen.com

With multiple new articles a day on various holistic health, fitness, nutrition, and spirituality topics, this website is a great resource for learning more about holistic wellness.

BalancedBabe.com

My personal blog features hundreds of free health-conscious recipe options, many of them plant-based, and other nutrition tips and tricks.

Gaia.com

This is a wonderful website that offers educational videos and streaming workshops to practice yoga, meditation, and spirituality.

TheHotline.org

The National Domestic Violence Hotline provides local resources and organizations for people experiencing domestic abuse. They also run a hotline to assist people in finding safety at 1-800-799-7233 (SAFE).

NCADV.org

The National Coalition Against Domestic Violence website lists numerous national hotlines for various types of abuse situations, from domestic abuse to child abuse.

Podcasts

The Ultimate Health Podcast

This podcast focuses on interviews with various wellness experts on topics like healthy eating, mindfulness, and more.

Nutrition Facts with Dr. Greger

Each episode is around 15 minutes long and provides easy-to-implement tips and tricks to healthy eating.

The Mindful Minute

This podcast revolves around discussions on meditation followed by guided meditations you can do at home.

Simplified With Sarah

My podcast provides free guided meditations and holistic health episodes that will further help you cultivate a natural lifestyle.

REFERENCES

Andrade, Ana M., Geoffrey W. Greene, and Kathleen J. Melanson. "Eating Slowly Led to Decreases in Energy Intake within Meals in Healthy Women." *Journal of the Academy of Nutrition and Dietics* 108, no. 7 (July 1, 2008): 1186–1191. doi.org/10.1016/j.jada .2008.04.026.

Apaydin, Eric A., Alicia R. Maher, Roberta Shanman, Marika S. Booth, Jeremy N. V. Miles, Melony E. Sorbero, and Susanne Hempel. "A Systematic Review of St. John's Wort for Major Depressive Disorder." *Systematic Reviews* 5, no. 1 (September 2, 2016). doi.org/10.1186/s13643-016-0325-2.

Bent, Stephen, Amy Padula, Dan Moore, Michael Patterson, and Wolf Mehling. "Valerian for Sleep: A Systematic Review and Meta-Analysis." *American Journal of Medicine* 119, no. 12 (December 1, 2006): 1005–1112. doi.org/10.1016 /j.amjmed.2006.02.026.

Berkman, L. F., and S. L. Syme. "Social Networks, Host Resistance, and Mortality: A Nine-Year Follow-up Study of Alameda County Residents." *American Journal of Epidemiology* 109, no. 2 (February 1, 1979): 186–204. doi.org/10.1093/oxfordjournals .aje.a112674.

Broadhouse, Kathryn M., Maria Fiatarone Singh, Chao Suo, Nicola Gates, Wei Wen, Henry Brodaty, Nidhi Jain et al. "Hippocampal Plasticity Underpins Long-Term Cognitive Gains from Resistance Exercise in MCI." *NeuroImage: Clinical* 25 (January 14, 2020): 102182. doi.org/10.1016/j.nicl.2020.102182.

Carr, Deborah, and Kristen W. Springer. "Advances in Families and Health Research in the 21st Century." *Journal of Marriage and Family* 72, no. 3 (June 18, 2010): 743–761. doi.org /10.1111/j.1741-3737.2010.00728.x.

Creswell, J. David, Janine M. Dutcher, William M. P. Klein, Peter R. Harris, and John M. Levine. "Self-Affirmation Improves Problem-Solving under Stress." *PLoS ONE* 8, no. 5 (May 1, 2013): e62593. doi.org/10.1371/journal.pone .0062593.

Fay, Bill. "Key Figures behind America's Consumer Debt." Debt.org. Accessed May 25, 2020. Debt.org/faqs/americans -in-debt.

Fißler, Maria, and Arnim Quante. "A Case Series on the Use of Lavendula Oil Capsules in Patients Suffering from Major Depressive Disorder and Symptoms of Psychomotor Agitation, Insomnia, and Anxiety." *Complementary Therapies in Medicine* 22, no. 1 (February 2014): 63–69. doi.org /10.1016/j.ctim.2013.11.008.

Gottlieb, Scott. "Mental Activity May Help Prevent Dementia." *BMJ* 326, no. 7404 (June 28, 2003): 1418. ncbi.nlm.nih .gov/pmc/articles/PMC1151037.

Harvard Health Publishing. "Preserve Your Muscle Mass." Harvard Health. Published February 19, 2016. health.harvard .edu/staying-healthy/preserve-your -muscle-mass.

Harvard Health Publishing. "Probiotics May Help Boost Mood and Cognitive Function." Harvard Health. Accessed June 14, 2020. health.harvard.edu /mind-and-mood/probiotics-may-help -boost-mood-and-cognitive-function.

Holt-Lunstad J., et al. "Social Relationships and Mortality Risk: A Meta-Analytic Review." *PLoS Medicine* 7, no. 7 (July 27, 2010). doi .org/10.1371/journal.pmed.1000316.

Josling, P. "Preventing the Common Cold with a Garlic Supplement: A Double-Blind, Placebo-Controlled Survey." *Advances in Therapy* 18, no. 4 (July 1, 2001): 189–193. doi.org /10.1007/BF02850113.

Kardan, Omid, Peter Gozdyra, Bratislav Misic, Faisal Moola, Lyle J. Palmer, Tomáš Paus, and Marc G. Berman. "Neighborhood Greenspace and Health in a Large Urban Center." *Scientific Reports* 5, no. 11610 (July 9, 2015). doi.org/10.1038/srep11610.

Kawai, Nobuhiro, Noriaki Sakai, Masashi Okuro, Sachie Karakawa, Yosuke Tsuney-oshi, Noriko Kawasaki, Tomoko Takeda, Makoto Bannai, and Seiji Nishino. "The Sleep-Promoting and Hypothermic Effects of Glycine Are Mediated by NMDA Receptors in the Suprachiasmatic Nucleus." *Neuropsychopharmacology* 40, no. 6 (December 23, 2014): 1405–1416. doi.org/10.1038/npp.2014.326.

Kunutsor, Setor Kwadzo, Tanjaniina Laukkanen, and Jari Antero Laukkanen. "Sauna Bathing Reduces the Risk of Respiratory Diseases: A Long-Term Prospective Cohort Study." *European Journal of Epidemiology* 32, no. 12

(September 13, 2017): 1107–1111. doi.org/10.1007/s10654-017-0311-6.

Levy, Becca R., Martin D. Slade, Suzanne R. Kunkel, and Stanislav V. Kasl. "Longevity Increased by Positive Self-Perceptions of Aging." *Journal of Personality and Social Psychology* 83, no. 2 (2002): 261–270. doi.org/10.1037/0022-3514.83.2.261.

Ludy, Mary-Jon, and Richard D. Mattes. "The Effects of Hedonically Acceptable Red Pepper Doses on Thermogenesis and Appetite." *Physiology & Behavior* 102, no. 3–4 (March 2011): 251–58. doi.org /10.1016/j.physbeh.2010.11.018.

Mischoulon, David. "Omega-3 Fatty Acids for Mood Disorders." Harvard Health Blog. Published August 3, 2018. health.harvard.edu/blog/omega -3-fatty-acids-for-mood-disorders -2018080314414.

Morita, E., S. Fukuda, J. Nagano, N. Hamajima, H. Yamamoto, Y. Iwai, T. Nakashima, H. Ohira, and T. Shirakawa. "Psychological Effects of Forest Environments on Healthy Adults: Shinrin-Yoku (Forest-Air Bathing, Walking) as a Possible Method of Stress Reduction." *Public Health* 121, no. 1 (January 2007): 54–63. doi .org/10.1016/j.puhe.2006.05.024.

Müller, Max. *India: What Can It Teach Us? A Course of Lectures Delivered before the University of Cambridge*. London: Longmans, Green, and Co., 1892. Accessed electronically: archive.org /details/indiawhatcanitte00mluoft.

Nystoriak, Matthew A., and Aruni Bhatnagar. "Cardiovascular Effects and Benefits of Exercise." *Frontiers in Cardiovascular Medicine* 5 (September 28, 2018): 135. doi.org/10.3389/fcvm .2018.00135.

Oschman, James, Gaetan Chevalier, and Richard Brown. "The Effects of Ground-ing (Earthing) on Inflammation, the Immune Response, Wound Healing, and Prevention and Treatment of Chronic Inflammatory and Autoimmune Diseases." *Journal of Inflammation Research* 2015, no. 8 (March 24, 2015): 83–96. doi.org/10.2147/JIR.S69656.

Park, Bum Jin, Yuko Tsunetsugu, Tamami Kasetani, Takahide Kagawa, and Yoshifumi Miyazaki. "The Physiological Effects of *Shinrin-Yoku* (Taking in the Forest Atmosphere or Forest Bathing): Evidence from Field Experiments in 24 Forests across Japan." *Environmental Health and Preventive Medicine* 15, no. 1 (May 2, 2009): 18–26. doi.org/10.1007 /s12199-009-0086-9.

Park, Denise C., Jennifer Lodi-Smith, Linda Drew, Sara Haber, Andrew Hebrank, Gérard N. Bischof, and Whitley Aamodt. "The Impact of Sustained Engagement on Cognitive Function in Older Adults." *Psychological Science* 25, no. 1 (November 8, 2013): 103–112. doi.org /10.1177/0956797613499592.

Park, Ui-Hyun, Hong-Suk Jeong, Eun-Young Jo, Taesun Park, Seung Kew Yoon, Eun-Joo Kim, Ji-Cheon Jeong, and Soo-Jong Um. "Piperine, a Component of Black Pepper, Inhibits Adipogenesis by Antagonizing PPARγ Activity in 3T3-L1 Cells." *Journal of Agricultural and Food Chemistry* 60, no. 15 (April 2, 2012): 3853–3860. doi.org/10.1021/jf204514a.

Peden, A. R., M. K. Rayens, L. A. Hall, and L. H. Beebe. "Preventing Depression in High-Risk College Women: A Report of an 18-Month Follow-Up." *Journal of American College Health* 49, no. 6 (2001): 299–306. doi.org /10.1080/07448480109596316.

Pieters, Huibrie C., Leilanie Ayala, Ariel Schneider, Nancy Wicks, Aimee Levine-Dickman, and Susan Clinton. "Gardening on a Psychiatric Inpatient Unit: Cultivating Recovery." *Archives of Psychiatric Nursing* 33, no. 1 (February 1, 2019): 57–64. doi.org /10.1016/j.apnu.2018.10.001.

Roundtable on Population Health Improvement, Board on Population Health and Public Health Practice, Institute of Medicine, Business Engagement in Building Healthy Communities: Workshop Summary. *Lessons from the Blue Zones®*. Washington, DC: National Academies Press, 2015. Access electronically: ncbi.nlm.nih.gov/books/NBK298903.

"Spirituality." Lexico Dictionaries, English. 2019. Lexico.com/en/definition /spirituality.

Tafet, G. E., V. P. Idoyaga-Vargas, D. P. Abulafia, J. M. Calandria, S. S. Roffman, A. Chiovetta, and M. Shinitzky. "Correlation between Cortisol Level and Serotonin Uptake in Patients with Chronic Stress and Depression." *Cognitive, Affective, & Behavioral Neuroscience* 1 (December 2001): 388–93. doi.org/10.3758/cabn.1.4.388.

Taylor-Piliae, Ruth E., and Brooke A. Finley. "Tai Chi Exercise for Psychological Well-Being among Adults with Cardiovascular Disease: A Systematic Review and Meta-Analysis." *European Journal of Cardiovascular Nursing* (June 9, 2020). doi.org/10.1177/1474515120926068.

Tang, Hongliang, Zhao Chen, Jun Pang, and Qiaoming Mo. "Treatment of Insomnia with Shujing Massage Therapy: A Randomized Controlled Trial." *Chinese*

Acupuncture & Moxibustion (translation) 35, no. 8 (August 2015): 816–818. pubmed.ncbi.nlm.nih.gov/26571900.

Thomas, Patricia A., Hui Liu, and Debra Umberson. "Family Relationships and Well-Being." *Innovation in Aging* 1, no. 3 (November 11, 2017). doi.org/10.1093/geroni/igx025.

University of East Anglia. "It's Official—Spending Time Outside Is Good for You." ScienceDaily. Published July 6, 2018. ScienceDaily.com/releases/2018/07/180706102842.htm.

University of Illinois College of Agricultural, Consumer, and Environmental Sciences. "Immune System May Be Pathway between Nature and Good Health." ScienceDaily. Published September 16, 2015. ScienceDaily.com/releases/2015/09/150916162120.htm.

Walker, William H., James C. Walton, A. Courtney DeVries, and Randy J. Nelson. "Circadian Rhythm Disruption and Mental Health. *Translational Psychiatry* 10, no. 28 (January 23, 2020). doi.org/10.1038/s41398-020-0694-0.

Willcox, B. J., D. C. Willcox, H. Todoriki, A. Fujiyoshi, K. Yano, Q. He, J. D. Curb, and M. Suzuki. "Caloric Restriction, the Traditional Okinawan Diet, and Healthy Aging: The Diet of the World's Longest-Lived People and Its Potential Impact on Morbidity and Life Span." *Annals of the New York Academy of Sciences* 1114, no. 1 (October 2007): 434–455. doi.org/10.1196/annals.1396.037.

Zaidel, Dahlia W. "Creativity, Brain, and Art: Biological and Neurological Considerations." *Frontiers in Human Neuroscience* 8 (June 2, 2014). doi.org/10.3389/fnhum.2014.00389.

Zakay-Rones, Z., E. Thom, T. Wollan, and J. Wadstein. "Randomized Study of the Efficacy and Safety of Oral Elderberry Extract in the Treatment of Influenza A and B Virus Infections." *Journal of International Medical Research* 32, no. 2 (March 1, 2004): 132–140. doi.org/10.1177/147323000403200205.

INDEX

////////////////////////////

hormone imbalance, alternative
treatments for, 86
hunger hormones, 66, 84
melatonin, 80, 85, 107, 108
weight-regulating hormones, 59, 83
Humanistic therapy, 30–31
Hydration, maintaining, 78
Hydrotherapy, 79

I

Ideal Daily Schedule templates, 42, 92, 124
Immune system
daily practices to boost, 78
home remedies, bolstering, 77, 86
immune-supporting nutrients
in food heroes, 63
intentional physical movement
as improving, 69
lifestyle tips, 79
outdoor time as beneficial for, 107
Insulin levels, 66, 83
Integrative therapy, 31
Intentionality
cognitive behavioral therapy as aiding, 30
commuting in an intentional way, 17
forest bathing with, 109
intention setting, 40, 90–91, 122
intentional movement, 69, 72
mindfulness and, 4, 7
in reframed thinking, 59
resources for living with intention, 128

J

Journaling
benefits of, 34
as a daily practice, 81

on family and culture of origin, 119
food journal, keeping, 68
intention setting, 40
personal mantra creation, 11
in quiet reflection space, 101, 102
Jung, Carl, 26

K

Kapha body type, 49, 51, 52, 54–55

L

Law of Attraction, 99
Loma Linda, California, 62

M

Magnesium, 58, 63, 64, 65, 84, 85
Mantras, 5, 7, 10–11
Marma point therapy, 75, 86
Massage
Ayurveda, as part of treatment
in, 49, 75
benefits of, 76, 86
bodywork, pondering the need for, 90
massage appointments, booking
as part of action plan, 91
self-massage, 72, 84
Matcha, 80
Meals. *See* Diet and nutrition
Meditation
Ayurveda, as a practice in, 49
balance, promoting, 55
bedtime, practicing prior to, 84, 105
daily practice of, 78
mantra and chanting meditations, 10–11
meditation app, 128
meditation podcasts, 130

R

Reframing, 24, 59
Reiki, 74, 86
Relationships
  archetypal pattern of, 26
  building and strengthening,
    111–112, 113–114, 115
  family relationships, 112–113, 116–117
  foundations of healthy
    relationships, 18–19
  maintaining healthy relationships, 22, 82
  sexual stress in relationships, 20–21
  unhealthy or harmful patterns,
    recognizing, 19–20
Restorative yoga, 71
Rhodiola, 80

S

Sacred space and time, creating,
  98, 101–102
Saint-John's-wort, 82
Sardinia, Italy, 61
Sauna bathing, 55, 78
Scent therapy, 55, 84, 85, 86, 90
Seated Body Scan meditation, 9
Self-care
  ancient systems of, 48
  designated spiritual space,
    establishing for, 105
  forms of, 20
  healer archetype and, 28
  naturopathy, as a focus of, 77
  self-care routines, developing, 59
  self-healing through home remedies, 86
  self-massage as a self-care practice, 84
  tai chi as a self-care modality, 72

Self-talk, 24, 31, 104
Sensory rituals, creating, 81
Shiatsu, 76, 86
Shoshin (beginner's mind), 5–6
Sleep
  avocado as promoting good sleep, 65
  circadian rhythm, supporting, 108, 110
  grounding as improving the
    quality of sleep, 109
  home remedies as improving
    sleep, 77, 86
  hormones as regulating, 56, 59
  kapha body type, sleep
    habits of, 51, 52, 55
  lifestyle tips to improve sleep, 80, 84, 85
  marma point therapy for
    sleep distress, 75
  meditation as helping to improve, 7
  self-inquiry into sleep habits, 90
Spiritual Wellness Plan template, 123
Stoicism, 6–7
Stress
  Ayurvedic response to, 49
  chronic stress, 29
  clutter as a stressor, 99
  cortisol as a stress hormone,
    71, 78, 80, 108, 110
  environmental stress, 17
  financial stress, 15–16
  journaling for stress relief, 81
  marma point therapy for high
    levels of stress, 75
  meditation, managing with,
    7, 13, 78, 108
  mindfulness, handling with, 15, 17, 21
  occupational stress, 14–15

podcasts regarding, 130
serving others as a wellness
    practice, 118, 119
sexual wellness, cultivating, 21
sleep, wellness practices
    improving, 90
spiritual wellness, setting
    intention for, 122
unique wellness blueprint,
    quiz to discover, 51
wellness plan, creating, 40, 41
Wellness Plan For My Mind
    template, 41
Whole foods, 66, 67, 68

ACKNOWLEDGMENTS

////////////////////////////

I'd like to acknowledge my mother who, from when I was young, was always experimenting with different homeopathic remedies and holistic modalities. Her interest in holistic health, spirituality, and meditation ignited my curiosity from a young age and led me to have a career path in this space! I'd also like to thank my father for being a strong source of faith in my life and always teaching me the importance of connecting with God through prayer and affirmations. If not for him, I would not have had the faith to follow my dreams.

Finally, I'd like to acknowledge my husband, who wholeheartedly supports every step I take in my career path and as a mother. He happily acts as my guinea pig, testing out all the new recipes, home remedies, and healing techniques I learn. With him as my partner I am proud to say I am elevated to always pursue my passions with him cheering me on.

ABOUT THE AUTHOR

////////////////////////////

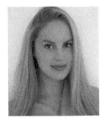

Sarah Baker is an internationally accredited meditation teacher, integrative and plant-based nutrition consultant, holistic health and mindset coach, Reiki practitioner, postpartum doula, and holistic health coach. She is the founder of SenseSanctuary.com, a virtual meditation and wellness studio and holistic health boutique, and BalancedBabe.com, an online platform with more than 800 articles, recipes, and homeopathic remedies. Sarah educates and shares her expertise with a wide audience as a health correspondent on various morning TV shows; through her first published book, *The Vegetarian Cookbook for Teens*; and on her podcast, *Simplified with Sarah*. You can learn more about Sarah on her Instagram @simplifiedwithsarah and at SarahNicoleBaker.com.